Pathology and Diagnosis of Gynecologic Diseases

Pathology and Diagnosis of Gynecologic Diseases

Editors

Cinzia Giacometti
Kathrin Ludwig

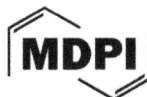

Basel • Beijing • Wuhan • Barcelona • Belgrade • Novi Sad • Cluj • Manchester

Editors

Cinzia Giacometti
Pathology Unit, Department
of Diagnostic Sciences, ULSS
6 Euganea
Padua, Italy

Kathrin Ludwig
Pathology Unit, Department
of Medicine, Azienda
Ospedaliera di Padova
Padua, Italy

Editorial Office
MDPI
St. Alban-Anlage 66
4052 Basel, Switzerland

This is a reprint of articles from the Special Issue published online in the open access journal *Diagnostics* (ISSN 2075-4418) (available at: https://www.mdpi.com/journal/diagnostics/special_issues/Gynecology_Pathology).

For citation purposes, cite each article independently as indicated on the article page online and as indicated below:

Lastname, A.A.; Lastname, B.B. Article Title. *Journal Name* **Year**, *Volume Number*, Page Range.

ISBN 978-3-0365-9800-0 (Hbk)
ISBN 978-3-0365-9801-7 (PDF)
doi.org/10.3390/books978-3-0365-9801-7

© 2024 by the authors. Articles in this book are Open Access and distributed under the Creative Commons Attribution (CC BY) license. The book as a whole is distributed by MDPI under the terms and conditions of the Creative Commons Attribution-NonCommercial-NoDerivs (CC BY-NC-ND) license.

Contents

Cinzia Giacometti and Kathrin Ludwig
Editorial on the Special Issue Titled "Pathology and Diagnosis of Gynecologic Diseases"
Reprinted from: *Diagnostics* **2023**, *13*, 3480, doi:10.3390/diagnostics13223480 1

**Alice Bergamini, Giorgia Mangili, Alessandro Ambrosi, Gianluca Taccagni,
Emanuela Rabaiotti, Luca Bocciolone, et al.**
Endometriosis-Related Ovarian Cancers: Evidence for a Dichotomy in the Histogenesis of the Two Associated Histotypes
Reprinted from: *Diagnostics* **2023**, *13*, 1425, doi:10.3390/diagnostics13081425 7

Jihee Sohn, Yurimi Lee and Hyun-Soo Kim
Endometrioid Carcinomas of the Ovaries and Endometrium Involving Endocervical Polyps: Comprehensive Clinicopathological Analyses
Reprinted from: *Diagnostics* **2022**, *12*, 2339, doi:10.3390/diagnostics12102339 17

**Tip Pongsuvareeyakul, Kanokkan Saipattranusorn, Kornkanok Sukpan,
Prapaporn Suprasert and Surapan Khunamornpong**
Clear-Cell Mesothelioma of Uterine Corpus: Diagnostic Challenges in Intraoperative Frozen Sections
Reprinted from: *Diagnostics* **2023**, *13*, 1119, doi:10.3390/diagnostics13061119 37

Chanyuan Li, Ting Deng, Junya Cao, Yun Zhou, Xiaolin Luo, Yanling Feng, et al.
Identifying ITGB2 as a Potential Prognostic Biomarker in Ovarian Cancer
Reprinted from: *Diagnostics* **2023**, *13*, 1169, doi:10.3390/diagnostics13061169 45

**Mayumi Kinoshita, Motoji Sawabe, Yurie Soejima, Makiko Naka Mieno, Tomio Arai and
Naoko Honma**
Gross Cystic Disease Fluid Protein-15 (GCDFP-15) Expression Characterizes Breast Mucinous Carcinomas in Older Women
Reprinted from: *Diagnostics* **2022**, *12*, 3129, doi:10.3390/diagnostics12123129 59

**Oana Gabriela Trifanescu, Raluca Alexandra Trifanescu, Radu Iulian Mitrica,
Diana Maria Bran, Georgia Luiza Serbanescu, Laurentiu Valcauan, et al.**
The Female Reproductive Tract Microbiome and Cancerogenesis: A Review Story of Bacteria, Hormones, and Disease
Reprinted from: *Diagnostics* **2023**, *13*, 877, doi:10.3390/diagnostics13050877 73

**Christoforos Kosmidis, Christina Sevva, Vasiliki Magra, Nikolaos Varsamis,
Charilaos Koulouris, Ioannis Charalampous, et al.**
HPV-Induced Anal and Peri-Anal Neoplasia, a Surgeon's Experience: 5-Year Case Series
Reprinted from: *Diagnostics* **2023**, *13*, 702, doi:10.3390/diagnostics13040702 87

**Suheyla Ekemen, Cem Comunoglu, Cavit Kerem Kayhan, Ebru Bilir, Ilkay Cavusoglu,
Nilay Etiler, et al.**
Endometrial Staining of CD56 (Uterine Natural Killer), BCL-6, and CD138 (Plasma Cells) Improve Diagnosis and Clinical Pregnancy Outcomes in Unexplained Infertility and Recurrent IVF Failures: Standardization of Diagnosis with Digital Pathology
Reprinted from: *Diagnostics* **2023**, *13*, 1557, doi:10.3390/diagnostics13091557 99

**Cinzia Giacometti, Kathrin Ludwig, Monica Guidi, Elvira Colantuono, Anna Coracina,
Marcello Rigano, et al.**
Gestational Diabetes—Placental Expression of Human Equilibrative Nucleoside Transporter 1 (hENT1): Is Delayed Villous Maturation an Adaptive Pattern?
Reprinted from: *Diagnostics* **2023**, *13*, 2034, doi:10.3390/diagnostics13122034 111

Hera Jung
Complete Hydatidiform Mole with Lung Metastasis and Coexisting Live Fetus: Unexpected Twin Pregnancy Mimicking Placenta Accreta
Reprinted from: *Diagnostics* **2023**, *13*, 2249, doi:10.3390/diagnostics13132249 . . . . **123**

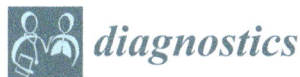

Editorial

Editorial on the Special Issue Titled "Pathology and Diagnosis of Gynecologic Diseases"

Cinzia Giacometti [1,*] and Kathrin Ludwig [2]

1 Pathology Unit, Department of Diagnostic Sciences, ULSS 6 Euganea, 35131 Padova, Italy
2 Pathology Unit, Department of Medicine, University of Padova, 35128 Padova, Italy; kathrin.ludwig@aopd.veneto.it
* Correspondence: cinzia.giacometti@aulss6.veneto.it

1. Introduction

In the medical and diagnostic daily routine, gynecologic diseases present many different scenarios. Benign lesions may mimic malignant ones, and vice versa; hormonal effects (either menstrual, pregnancy, or therapy-related) may alter normal histology and create artifacts; systemic diseases, such as diabetes and connective tissue diseases, may influence the hormonal status and affect placentation and gestation; genetic imbalance (BRCA, *p53*, mismatch repair protein deficiency—dMMR) can cause breast, endometrial, and ovary cancer [1–4]. This female "cosmos," in which so much is interconnected and happens due to something else, is complex, and diagnostic challenges, tricky differential diagnoses, and pitfalls are routinely encountered. For instance, in gynecologic pathology, the correlation between benign and malignant diseases in gynecologic pathology is well-described, with some overlap in ovarian endometrial cancer and endometriosis. Studies have shown that different malignant degeneration pathways can lead to the development of endometriosis-associated ovarian tumors of the endometrioid and clear cell histotypes [5,6]. In gynecologic pathology, benign diseases that can increase the risk of malignant disease and a variety of synchronous and multiple cancers are often encountered [7,8].

Researchers are still searching for new biomarkers to accurately predict common gynecologic tumors' prognosis. For instance, there is a need for novel prognostic biomarkers to improve immunotherapy, such as ITGB2 in ovarian cancer. Despite significant advancements in immunotherapy, patients with epithelial ovarian cancer still respond poorly to it; this could be due to immunosuppression and the high heterogeneity of the disease. Therefore, more research needs to be conducted to understand the molecular mechanisms in the ovarian cancer tumor immune microenvironment and develop new therapies that can effectively heat the "cold" ovarian cancer and enhance the clinical efficacy of immunotherapy [9,10].

Female genital cancer can develop due to various factors, such as viruses, bacteria, and hormonal and genetic imbalances. In recent years, research has shown that the microbiome also plays a significant role in cancer development; additionally, HPV infection increases the risk of developing squamous cell carcinoma in the skin and mucous membranes [11–14].

Gynecologic pathology encompasses neoplastic diseases and pregnancy-related pathology, a peculiar field; this includes pre-implantation disease, which has gained significant importance due to the wider use of in vitro fertilization [IVF] techniques [15–17]. But also, during pregnancy, various diseases can endanger the health of both the fetus and the mother. Some examples include gestational diabetes, which can disrupt normal placental function [18–20], and extremely rare but aggressive diseases, such as complete hydatidiform mole [21,22].

Citation: Giacometti, C.; Ludwig, K. Editorial on the Special Issue Titled "Pathology and Diagnosis of Gynecologic Diseases". *Diagnostics* **2023**, *13*, 3480. https://doi.org/10.3390/diagnostics13223480

Received: 1 October 2023
Accepted: 16 November 2023
Published: 20 November 2023

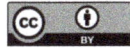

Copyright: © 2023 by the authors. Licensee MDPI, Basel, Switzerland. This article is an open access article distributed under the terms and conditions of the Creative Commons Attribution (CC BY) license (https://creativecommons.org/licenses/by/4.0/).

2. An Overview of Published Articles

Bergamini et al. (Contributor 1) compare data from patients affected by endometriosis-associated ovarian tumors of the endometrioid and clear cell histotypes to investigate the hypothesis of a dichotomy in the histogenesis of these tumors. The study analyzed clinical data and tumor characteristics of 48 patients who were diagnosed with either pure, clear cell ovarian cancer or mixed endometrioid-clear cell ovarian cancer arising from endometriosis (or endometriosis-associated endometrioid ovarian cancer). The exact pathways that lead to the development of cancer from endometriosis are not yet fully understood. However, it is known that the development of ovarian cancer in women with endometriosis is a complex process that involves multiple steps. It begins with forming a precursor lesion, such as atypical endometriosis, which contains certain genetic and epigenetic mutations. Over time, these changes accumulate and are further compounded by the inflammatory, hyperestrogenic environment and oxidative stress in the endometriotic lesion, ultimately leading to the development of cancer. A particular subtype of endometriosis-associated ovarian cancer appears to develop slowly within an endometriotic cyst; this represents a subset of diseases where ultrasound could be useful in the early detection of malignant degeneration.

Sohn et al. (Contributor 2) analyzed tumors coexisting with endocervical polyps (ECPs) and studied the clinicopathological characteristics of ovarian and endometrial ECs involving ECPs. The study identified 429 ECPs, most associated with premalignant or malignant lesions in the uterine cervix, endometrium, and ovaries. No evidence of benign endometriosis, endometrial hyperplasia without atypia, or atypical hyperplasia/endometrial intraepithelial neoplasm within ECPs or the adjacent endocervical tissue was noted. According to the results, the involvement of ECPs by EC may have been due to an implantation metastasis from the ovarian or endometrial EC. The pathogenic mechanism of ECP involvement may have been implantation metastasis via transtubal and trans-endometrial cavity migration.

The article by Pongsuvareeyakul et al. (Contributor 3) reinforces the concept that determining the type and source of metastatic tumors is a crucial and potentially difficult task in pathology because it affects clinical decision-making and management of patients, as it may occur during an intraoperative exam when the site of origin of a clear cell tumor can pose an unpredictable diagnostic challenge. The authors presented a case of clear-cell mesothelioma, which originated in the uterine serosa and was initially misdiagnosed as clear-cell adenocarcinoma in the intraoperative frozen section. The tumor showed diffuse tubulocystic spaces of variable size lined by clear cells with moderate nuclear atypia. Immunohistochemical staining confirmed the diagnosis of clear-cell mesothelioma. This variant of epithelioid mesothelioma is an extremely rare neoplasm of the peritoneum and shares histomorphologic features overlapping with many other tumors, including carcinomas and non-epithelial neoplasms. Diagnosing peritoneal clear-cell mesothelioma is not always straightforward, despite known immunohistochemistry (IHC) markers. Due to its rarity, it may be easily confused with other clear-cell neoplasms, especially in intraoperative frozen sections. However, recognizing this rare entity is essential as the diagnosis could significantly affect the management considerations. The authors concluded that using an IHC panel judiciously can help distinguish this tumor from other mimickers.

Li, C, and colleagues (Contributor 4) conducted an integrated bioinformatic analysis to identify genes related to ovarian tumorigenesis and their immune characteristics in the ovarian cancer microenvironment. They filtered 332 differentially expressed genes from a database and identified 10 upregulated hub genes closely associated with ovarian tumorigenesis. The team proceeded to perform a survival and immune infiltration analysis that demonstrated that the upregulation of five candidate genes, ITGB2, VEGFA, CLDN4, OCLN, and SPP1, were correlated with unfavorable clinical outcomes and increased immune cell infiltration in ovarian cancer. Among these genes, ITGB2 correlated most with various immune cell infiltrations and strongly correlated with significant M2 macrophage infiltration while having a moderate correlation with CD4+/CD8+ T cells and B cells. This characteristic explains why ITGB2's high expression was accompanied by immune activation but did not reverse carcinogenesis. Additionally, Western blotting and immunohistochemistry confirmed that ITGB2 was over-expressed in ovarian cancer tissues, primarily in the cytoplasm. In summary, ITGB2 may be a prognostic immunomarker for ovarian cancer patients.

The study by Kinoshita et al. (Contributor 5) explores the predominant histological subtype of breast mucinous carcinoma in older women, which is type B (hypercellular), while in younger women, it is type A (hypocellular). The characteristics of mucinous carcinomas of the same histological subtype may differ between older and younger women. The study aimed to systematically clarify mucinous carcinomas' pathological and immunohistochemical features. Gross cystic disease fluid protein-15 (GCDFP-15) and eight other markers were used for immunostaining. The results showed that GCDFP-15 positivity was significantly higher in the older group compared to the younger group. Therefore, this study suggests that GCDFP-15 expression characterizes mucinous carcinomas in older women.

In the review by Trifanescu et al. (Contributor 6), the authors highlighted how the vagina harbors the highest number of bacteria, with a healthy profile dominated by Lactobacillus spp. On the other hand, the upper reproductive tract of females (consisting of the uterus, Fallopian tubes, and ovaries) has only a minimal number of bacteria. Although it was previously believed to be sterile, recent research has revealed the presence of a small microbiota in this region, with ongoing debates on whether it is a normal or pathological occurrence. It is noteworthy that the composition of the female reproductive tract's microbiota is significantly influenced by estrogen levels. Increasingly, research suggests a correlation between the microbiome of the female reproductive tract and the development of gynecological cancers.

Kosmidis and colleagues (Contributor 7) discuss a series of cases of neoplasia in the anal and perianal region, highlighting the ongoing debate about whether young males and adult males should be vaccinated against HPV. Currently, there are no official guidelines regarding widespread vaccination for males or screening for anal SCC or HSIL (high-grade squamous intraepithelial lesion).

In their article, Ekemen et al. (Contributor 8) demonstrate the range of diagnostic tools available for predicting the outcome of IVF with the help of digital pathology. The authors explained how, in unexplained infertility and recurrent IVF failure cases, plasmacellular chronic endometritis and CD56 elevation (an increase in uterine NK cells) can be detected through three immunohistochemical stains; this helps in providing a specific treatment. This study also found that BCL-6 correlated well with CD56 positivity, even better than CD56 immunopositivity alone. Additionally, as BCL-6 positivity is associated with pelvic endometriosis, immunostaining of curettage material can allow for an easy diagnosis and protect individuals from more invasive interventions. However, further studies are required to evaluate BCL-6's positivity in the endometrium.

Giacometti et al.'s (Contributor 9) research investigated the hypothesis that the absence or low expression of hENT1 in endothelial cells of all GDMd placentas could indicate a potential role in microvascular adaptive mechanisms. Due to the complex nature of the placental microenvironment, various pathways and metabolic mechanisms are likely to be affected by the alterations found at both cellular and phenotypic levels in GDM.

The article by Jung et al. (Contributor 10) reported an unusual case of placenta accreta, which was later determined to be an invasive hydatidiform mole. Unfortunately, it was not initially diagnosed as such. After radiologic examination, metastatic lung lesions were discovered, and the patient underwent six cycles of methotrexate administered at two-week intervals. The authors present this unexpected choriocarcinoma's clinical and pathological characteristics with pulmonary metastasis, compare it to existing literature, and highlight the importance of thorough pathological examination.

3. Conclusions

The compilation of articles in this Special Issue on gynecologic pathology covers a wide range of research, reflecting the richness of this field. The studies adopted different methodologies, including observational approaches, such as case studies, molecular biology, and artificial intelligence. It is worth noting that the articles published in this Special Issue are from around the world, highlighting the relevance and importance of this publication. It offers readers a chance to discover research focused on extra-national contexts, which allows for a more complete understanding of the research field of gynecologic pathology.

Author Contributions: Conceptualization, C.G.; writing—original draft preparation, C.G.; writing—review and editing, C.G. and K.L. All authors have read and agreed to the published version of the manuscript.

Funding: This research received no external funding.

Conflicts of Interest: The authors declare no conflict of interest.

List of Contributions

1. Bergamini, A.; Mangili, G.; Ambrosi, A.; Taccagni, G.; Rabaiotti, E.; Bocciolone, L.; Candotti, G.; Cioffi, R.; Pella, F.; Sabetta, G.; et al. Endometriosis-Related Ovarian Cancers: Evidence for a Dichotomy in the Histogenesis of the Two Associated Histotypes. *Diagnostics* **2023**, *13*, 1425. https://doi.org/10.3390/diagnostics13081425.
2. Sohn, J.; Lee, Y.; Kim, H. Endometrioid Carcinomas of the Ovaries and Endometrium Involving Endocervical Polyps: Comprehensive Clinicopathological Analyses. *Diagnostics* **2022**, *12*, 2339. https://doi.org/10.3390/diagnostics12102339.
3. Pongsuvareeyakul, T.; Saipattranusorn, K.; Sukpan, K.; Suprasert, P.; Khunamornpong, S. Clear-Cell Mesothelioma of Uterine Corpus: Diagnostic Challenges in Intraoperative Frozen Sections. *Diagnostics* **2023**, *13*, 1119. https://doi.org/10.3390/diagnostics13061119.
4. Li, C.; Deng, T.; Cao, J.; Zhou, Y.; Luo, X.; Feng, Y.; Huang, H.; Liu, J. Identifying ITGB2 as a Potential Prognostic Biomarker in Ovarian Cancer. *Diagnostics* **2023**, *13*, 1169. https://doi.org/10.3390/diagnostics13061169.
5. Kinoshita, M.; Sawabe, M.; Soejima, Y.; Mieno, M.; Arai, T.; Honma, N. Gross Cystic Disease Fluid Protein-15 [GCDFP-15] Expression Characterizes Breast Mucinous Carcinomas in Older Women. *Diagnostics* **2022**, *12*, 3129. https://doi.org/10.3390/diagnostics12123129.
6. Trifanescu, O.; Trifanescu, R.; Mitrica, R.; Bran, D.; Serbanescu, G.; Valcauan, L.; Marinescu, S.; Gales, L.; Tanase, B.; Anghel, R. The Female Reproductive Tract Microbiome and Cancerogenesis: A Review Story of Bacteria, Hormones, and Disease. *Diagnostics* **2023**, *13*, 877 https://doi.org/10.3390/diagnostics13050877.
7. Kosmidis, C.; Sevva, C.; Magra, V.; Varsamis, N.; Koulouris, C.; Charalampous, I.; Papadopoulos, K.; Roulia, P.; Dagher, M.; Theodorou, V.; et al. HPV-Induced Anal and Perianal Neoplasia, a Surgeon's Experience: 5-Year Case Series. *Diagnostics* **2023**, *13*, 702. https://doi.org/10.3390/diagnostics13040702.
8. Ekemen, S.; Comunoglu, C.; Kayhan, C.; Bilir, E.; Cavusoglu, I.; Etiler, N.; Bilgi, S.; Ince, U.; Coban, C.; Erden, H. Endometrial Staining of CD56 [Uterine Natural Killer], BCL-6, and CD138 [Plasma Cells] Improve Diagnosis and Clinical Pregnancy Outcomes in Unexplained Infertility and Recurrent IVF Failures: Standardization of Diagnosis with Digital Pathology. *Diagnostics* **2023**, *13*, 1557. https://doi.org/10.3390/diagnostics13091557.
9. Giacometti, C.; Ludwig, K.; Guidi, M.; Colantuono, E.; Coracina, A.; Rigano, M.; Cassaro, M.; Ambrosi, A. Gestational Diabetes—Placental Expression of Human Equilibrative Nucleoside Transporter 1 [hENT1]: Is Delayed Villous Maturation an Adaptive Pattern? *Diagnostics* **2023**, *13*, 2034. https://doi.org/10.3390/diagnostics13122034.
10. Jung, H. Complete Hydatidiform Mole with Lung Metastasis and Coexisting Live Fetus: Unexpected Twin Pregnancy Mimicking Placenta Accreta. *Diagnostics* **2023**, *13*, 2249. https://doi.org/10.3390/diagnostics13132249.

References

1. Chen, H.; Hu, X.; Wang, D.; Wang, Y.; Yu, Y.; Yao, H. Association of PIK3CA mutation with outcomes in HER2-positive breast cancer treated with anti-HER2 therapy: A meta-analysis and bioinformatic analysis of TCGA-BRCA data. *Transl. Oncol.* **2023**, *37*, 101738. [CrossRef] [PubMed]
2. Hynes, J.; Dawson, L.; Seal, M.; Green, J.; Woods, M.; Etchegary, H. "There should be one spot that you can go:" BRCA mutation carriers' perspectives on cancer risk management and a hereditary cancer registry. *J. Community Genet.* **2023**. [CrossRef] [PubMed]

3. Matsumoto, N.; Manrai, P.; Rottmann, D.; Wu, X.; Assem, H.; Hui, P.; Buza, N. Correlative Assessment of p53 Immunostaining Patterns and TP53 Mutation Status by Next-Generation Sequencing in High-Grade Endometrial Carcinomas. *Int. J. Gynecol. Pathol.* **2023**, *42*, 567–575. [CrossRef]
4. Saleh, A.; Perets, R. Mutated p53 in HGSC-From a Common Mutation to a Target for Therapy. *Cancers* **2021**, *13*, 3465. [CrossRef]
5. Beddows, I.; Fan, H.; Heinze, K.; Johnson, B.K.; Leonova, A.; Senz, J.; Djirackor, S.; Cho, K.R.; Pearce, C.L.; Huntsman, D.G.; et al. Cell state of origin impacts development of distinct endometriosis-related ovarian carcinoma histotypes. *Cancer Res.* **2023**. [CrossRef]
6. Addante, F.; Travaglino, A.; Arciuolo, D.; Fulgione, C.; Raffone, A.; Santoro, A.; Zannoni, G.F. Phenotypical plasticity of endometriosis-related ovarian neoplasms. *Virchows Arch.* **2023**. [CrossRef] [PubMed]
7. Yumisashi, R.; Saito, R.; Togami, S.; Kobayashi, Y.; Kitazono, I.; Tanimoto, A.; Kobayashi, H. Molecular biological analysis revealed a case of synchronous endometrial and ovarian cancer with different histological grade as metastatic ovarian cancer from endometrial cancer: Case report and review of literature. *J. Obstet. Gynaecol. Res.* **2023**, *11*, 2766–2770. [CrossRef]
8. Simion, L.; Chitoran, E.; Cirimbei, C.; Stefan, D.C.; Neicu, A.; Tanase, B.; Ionescu, S.O.; Luca, D.C.; Gales, L.; Gheorghe, A.S.; et al. A Decade of Therapeutic Challenges in Synchronous Gynecological Cancers from the Bucharest Oncological Institute. *Diagnostics* **2023**, *13*, 2069. [CrossRef]
9. Zhang, Y.; Guo, M.; Wang, L.; Weng, S.; Xu, H.; Ren, Y.; Liu, L.; Guo, C.; Cheng, Q.; Luo, P.; et al. A tumor-infiltrating immune cells-related pseudogenes signature based on machine-learning predicts outcomes and immunotherapy responses in ovarian cancer. *Cell Signal.* **2023**, *111*, 110879. [CrossRef]
10. Wang, R.; Du, X.; Zhi, Y. Screening of Critical Genes Involved in Metastasis and Prognosis of High-Grade Serous Ovarian Cancer by Gene Expression Profile Data. *J. Comput. Biol.* **2020**, *27*, 1104–1114. [CrossRef]
11. Li, X.; Wu, J.; Wu, Y.; Duan, Z.; Luo, M.; Li, L.; Li, S.; Jia, Y. Imbalance of Vaginal Microbiota and Immunity: Two Main Accomplices of Cervical Cancer in Chinese Women. *Int. J. Womens Health* **2023**, *15*, 987–1002. [CrossRef] [PubMed]
12. Barczynski, B.; Fraszczak, K.; Grywalska, E.; Kotarski, J.; Korona-Glowniak, I. Vaginal and Cervical Microbiota Composition in Patients with Endometrial Cancer. *Int. J. Mol. Sci.* **2023**, *24*, 8266. [CrossRef]
13. Sharifian, K.; Shoja, Z.; Jalilvand, S. The interplay between human papillomavirus and vaginal microbiota in cervical cancer development. *Virol. J.* **2023**, *20*, 73. [CrossRef]
14. Bowden, S.J.; Doulgeraki, T.; Bouras, E.; Markozannes, G.; Athanasiou, A.; Grout-Smith, H.; Kechagias, K.S.; Ellis, L.B.; Zuber, V.; Chadeau-Hyam, M.; et al. Risk factors for human papillomavirus infection, cervical intraepithelial neoplasia and cervical cancer: An umbrella review and follow-up Mendelian randomisation studies. *BMC Med.* **2023**, *21*, 274. [CrossRef] [PubMed]
15. Kanter, J.; Gordon, S.M.; Mani, S.; Sokalska, A.; Park, J.Y.; Senapati, S.; Huh, D.D.; Mainigi, M. Hormonal stimulation reduces numbers and impairs function of human uterine natural killer cells during implantation. *Hum. Reprod.* **2023**, *38*, 1047–1059. [CrossRef]
16. Dons Koi, B.V.; Osypchuk, D.V.; Baksheev, S.M.; Sudoma, I.O.; Goncharova, Y.O.; Palyha, I.E.; Sirenko, V.Y.; Khazhylenko, K.G.; Onyshchuk, O.; Anoshko, Y.; et al. A blinded multicenter investigation: Accentuated NK lymphocyte CD335 (NKp46) expression predicts reproductive failures after IVF. *Immunol. Lett.* **2022**, *251–252*, 47–55. [CrossRef] [PubMed]
17. Scarpellini, F.; Sbracia, M. Modification of peripheral Treg and CD56(bright)NK levels in RIF women after egg donation, treated with GM-CSF or placebo. *J. Reprod. Immunol.* **2023**, *158*, 103983. [CrossRef] [PubMed]
18. Giacometti, C.; Ludwig, K.; Guidi, M.; Colantuono, E.; Coracina, A.; Rigano, M.; Cassaro, M.; Ambrosi, A. Gestational Diabetes-Placental Expression of Human Equilibrative Nucleoside Transporter 1 (hENT1): Is Delayed Villous Maturation an Adaptive Pattern? *Diagnostics* **2023**, *13*, 2034. [CrossRef]
19. Diniz, M.S.; Hiden, U.; Falcao-Pires, I.; Oliveira, P.J.; Sobrevia, L.; Pereira, S.P. Fetoplacental endothelial dysfunction in gestational diabetes mellitus and maternal obesity: A potential threat for programming cardiovascular disease. *Biochim. Biophys. Acta Mol. Basis Dis.* **2023**, *1869*, 166834. [CrossRef]
20. Fato, B.R.; Beard, S.; Binder, N.K.; Pritchard, N.; Kaitu'u-Lino, T.J.; de Alwis, N.; Hannan, N.J. The Regulation of Endothelin-1 in Pregnancies Complicated by Gestational Diabetes: Uncovering the Vascular Effects of Insulin. *Biomedicines* **2023**, *11*, 2660. [CrossRef]
21. Wang, G.; Cui, H.; Chen, X. A complete hydatidiform mole and coexisting viable fetus in a twin pregnancy: A case report with literature review. *J. Matern. Fetal Neonatal Med.* **2023**, *36*, 2183746. [CrossRef] [PubMed]
22. Libretti, A.; Longo, D.; Faiola, S.; De Pedrini, A.; Troia, L.; Remorgida, V. A twin pregnancy with partial hydatidiform mole and a coexisting normal fetus delivered at term: A case report and literature review. *Case Rep. Womens Health* **2023**, *39*, e00544. [CrossRef] [PubMed]

Disclaimer/Publisher's Note: The statements, opinions and data contained in all publications are solely those of the individual author(s) and contributor(s) and not of MDPI and/or the editor(s). MDPI and/or the editor(s) disclaim responsibility for any injury to people or property resulting from any ideas, methods, instructions or products referred to in the content.

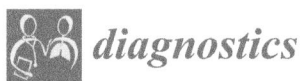

Article

Endometriosis-Related Ovarian Cancers: Evidence for a Dichotomy in the Histogenesis of the Two Associated Histotypes

Alice Bergamini [1,2,*], Giorgia Mangili [1], Alessandro Ambrosi [2], Gianluca Taccagni [3], Emanuela Rabaiotti [1], Luca Bocciolone [1], Giorgio Candotti [1], Raffaella Cioffi [1,2], Francesca Pella [1], Giulia Sabetta [1,2], Costanza Saponaro [1,2] and Massimo Candiani [1,2]

1 Obstetrics and Gynecology Unit, IRCCS San Raffaele Scientific Institute, 20132 Milan, Italy
2 Faculty of Medicine and Surgery, Vita-Salute San Raffaele University, Via Olgettina 58, 20132 Milan, Italy
3 Surgical Pathology Unit, IRCCS San Raffaele Scientific Institute, 20132 Milan, Italy
* Correspondence: bergamini.alice@hsr.it

Abstract: Evidence indicates that different pathways of malignant degeneration underlie the development of endometriosis-associated ovarian tumors of endometrioid and clear cell histotypes. The aim of this study was to compare data from patients affected by these two histotypes to investigate the hypothesis of a dichotomy in the histogenesis of these tumors. Clinical data and tumor characteristics of 48 patients who were diagnosed with either pure clear cell ovarian cancer and mixed endometrioid–clear cell ovarian cancer arising from endometriosis (ECC, n = 22) or endometriosis-associated endometrioid ovarian cancer (EAEOC, n = 26) were compared. A previous diagnosis of endometriosis was detected more frequently in the ECC group (32% vs. 4%, p = 0.01). The incidence of bilaterality was significantly higher in the EAOEC group (35% vs. 5%, p = 0.01) as well as a solid/cystic rate at gross pathology (57.7 ± 7.9% vs. 30.9 ± 7.5%, p = 0.02). Patients with ECC had a more advanced disease stage (41% vs. 15%; p = 0.04). A synchronous endometrial carcinoma was detected in 38% of EAEOC patients. A comparison of the International Federation of Gynecology and Obstetrics (FIGO) stage at diagnosis showed a significantly decreasing trend for ECC compared to EAEOC (p = 0.02). These findings support the hypothesis that the origin, clinical behavior and relationship with endometriosis might be different for these histotypes. ECC, unlike EAEOC, seems to develop within an endometriotic cyst, thus representing a window of possibility for ultrasound-based early diagnosis.

Keywords: ovarian cancer; endometrioid ovarian cancer; clear cell ovarian cancer; endometriosis; carcinogenesis

Citation: Bergamini, A.; Mangili, G.; Ambrosi, A.; Taccagni, G.; Rabaiotti, E.; Bocciolone, L.; Candotti, G.; Cioffi, R.; Pella, F.; Sabetta, G.; et al. Endometriosis-Related Ovarian Cancers: Evidence for a Dichotomy in the Histogenesis of the Two Associated Histotypes. *Diagnostics* 2023, *13*, 1425. https://doi.org/10.3390/diagnostics13081425

Academic Editor: Frediano Inzani

Received: 27 February 2023
Revised: 31 March 2023
Accepted: 11 April 2023
Published: 15 April 2023

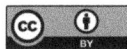

Copyright: © 2023 by the authors. Licensee MDPI, Basel, Switzerland. This article is an open access article distributed under the terms and conditions of the Creative Commons Attribution (CC BY) license (https://creativecommons.org/licenses/by/4.0/).

1. Introduction

Endometriosis is an estrogen-dependent chronic and progressive inflammatory disease, which affects 10% of all women of reproductive age in the world, equating to 190 million women worldwide [1–3]. It is characterized by the presence of extra-uterine, functionally active, endometrial tissue, represented by stroma and glands, which can be found mostly in the pelvic cavity, ovaries, fallopian tubes, sigmoid colon, appendix, upper abdomen and in other sites such as the lungs [4,5]. In particular, in 44% of cases, the ovaries are the site of endometriosis, with an endometriotic cyst defined as ovarian endometrioma [6]. The latter is evident in ultrasound examination as a unilocular cyst with homogeneous low-level echogenicity defined ground glass and absent to moderate vascularization [7]. From a molecular point of view, endometriosis is characterized by molecular abnormalities such as a loss of AT Rich Interactive Domain 1A (*ARID1A*) function, Phosphatase and Tensin homolog (*PTEN*) inactivation, Phosphatidylinositol-4,5-Bisphosphate 3-Kinase Catalytic Subunit Alpha (*PIK3CA*), Catenin Beta 1 (*CTNNB1*) and Kirsten Rat Sarcoma Viral oncogene homolog (*KRAS*) activation [6]. However, the etiology of this disease is still enigmatic. Several hypotheses have been proposed since 1870 and the most likely explanation is the retrograde menstruation theory. Additional postulated mechanisms include celomic metaplasia, lymphatic and vascular metastasis, endometrial stem cell implantation and abnormal residue of embryonic Mullerian tissue [8].

Endometriosis is a benign disease, but it shares some characteristics with cancer, such as local and distant invasion, resistance to apoptosis, recurrence, angiogenesis, damage to target organs and stimulation of the inflammatory system [9–14]. In particular, the real precursor of ovarian cancer is represented by atypical endometriosis which is seen in 60–80% of ovarian cancers that result from endometriosis [2,4].In addition, the most common mutations in atypical endometriosis affect *ARID1A*, *PIK3CA*, genes coding for estrogen and progestogen receptors, *KRAS* and *PTEN* [2].

The association between endometriosis and ovarian cancer was initially described in 1925 by Sampson, and then, it was confirmed by Scott in 1953, who observed that benign endometriosis may be present in proximity to ovarian cancer [2]. In particular, many studies confirm that the histotypes of epithelial ovarian cancer that are most closely related to endometriosis are endometrioid tumors and clear cell carcinoma [15,16]. In fact, these types have mutations in common with endometriosis, such as *PTEN*, *PIK3CA*, *KRAS* and *ARID1A* [15–17].

Sarria-Santamera and colleagues highlighted that endometriosis is correlated with a 2.66-fold greater risk of ovarian cancer, compared to the general population [18]. In addition, it has been estimated that the lifetime risk of ovarian cancer in women with endometriosis is 2.5% [1].

In a recent systematic review and meta-analysis by Kvaskoff and collaborators, it was estimated that those with clear cell and endometrioid histotypes had a greater risk of endometriosis, equal to 3.4-fold and 2.3-fold, respectively [9]. In particular, endometriosis is observed in 21–51% of women with clear cell ovarian cancer (CC) (odds ratio OR = 3.05) and in 23–43% of patients with endometrioid ovarian cancer (EOC) (OR = 2.04) [19]. Therefore, about one-third of all endometrioid and clear cell histotypes are estimated to arise from endometriosis; however, the mechanisms underlying the cancerogenesis of each subtype are not completely clear [19]. There is an increasing body of evidence suggesting that clear cell histotypes may arise from pre-existing endometriosis derived from retrograde menstruation, while endometrioid cancer derived from ovarian Mullerian metaplasia [20], with different pathways of malignant degeneration and different precursors, might be involved in the development of the two endometriosis-associated histotypes. In a very interesting paper, Kajihara and coworkers hypothesized a potential dichotomy in their histogenesis, suggesting that clear cell ovarian cancers which are associated with endometriosis may arise from pre-existing endometriosis derived from retrograde menstruation, whereas ovarian Mullerian metaplasia might be the initial event in the development of endometriosis-associated endometrioid cancers. Very few clinical studies have provided evidence forthe theory that for these two histotypes, the clinical behavior, prognosis and, most importantly, the origin and relation to endometriosis, might be different [20]. To the best of our knowledge, there are no studies which have specifically assessed this issue. The main reason is that, in several clinical series, these two histologies are often considered as a single entity, which are referred to as "endometriosis-associated ovarian tumors" [6]. This, together with the lack of adherence to the criteria for the pathological diagnosis of endometriosis-associated endometrioid ovarian tumors, as originally described by Sampson and Scott [21,22], might have prevented the correct identification of the study population. Finally, clinical studies addressing this area have, in general, compared characteristics of histotype-specific tumors which are associated, or are not associated, with endometriosis and not between endometriosis-associated cancers of different histotypes [9,23].

As a matter of fact, in two previous studies, our group separately analyzed these two histotypes, comparing endometrioid and clear cell carcinomas which were associated, or were not associated, with endometriosis [24,25]. In the first study considering endometrioid histology, we showed that compared to patients without endometriosis, women with endometriosis-associated endometrioid ovarian cancer were significantly younger at diagnosis, had a lower disease stage and had a less prevalent high-grade tumor. Interestingly, the rate of synchronous endometrial cancer was significantly higher in this group [24]. In the second study considering clear cell histology, patients with tumors arising from endometriosis were significantly younger, more frequently had a unilateral involvement and had a lower prevalence of ascites as the presenting symptom. No difference between the two groups was found for the International Federation of Gynecology and Obstetrics (FIGO) stage, laterality or the presence of a synchronous endometrial malignancy [25].

The aim of the present study was to clinically compare clinical data and tumor characteristics of patients affected by ovarian tumors of different histotypes which were associated with endometriosis, in order to verify the hypothesis supporting a dichotomy in the histogenesis of endometriosis-associated ovarian carcinomas, thus potentially offering interesting and novel clinical insights regarding this issue.

2. Materials and Methods

This was a retrospective study of 48 cases of ovarian tumors strictly associated with endometriosis, which were diagnosed and consecutively treated at the Obstetrics and Gynecology Unit of the Scientific Institute San Raffaele in Milan, Italy, between 1995 and 2016. Ethical approval was obtained from the San Raffaele Institute Ethics Board. All patients with a primary diagnosis of either pure clear cell ovarian cancer and mixed endometrioid–clear cell ovarian cancer strictly arising from endometriosis (ECC), or with endometriosis-associated endometrioid ovarian cancer (EAEOC), were included in the study. Patients whose diagnosis was made elsewhere were excluded. The definition of endometriosis arising from ovarian cancer was given according to Sampson's [21] and Scott's criteria [22], which included: (1) the coexistence of carcinoma and endometriosis in the same ovary; (2) the presence of tissue similar to endometrial stroma surrounding characteristic epithelial glands; (3) the exclusion of a metastatic tumor to the ovary and (4) the presence of benign endometriosis histologically contiguous with the malignant tissue. Patients with clear cell carcinoma associated with, but not arising from, endometriosis were excluded (Figure 1).

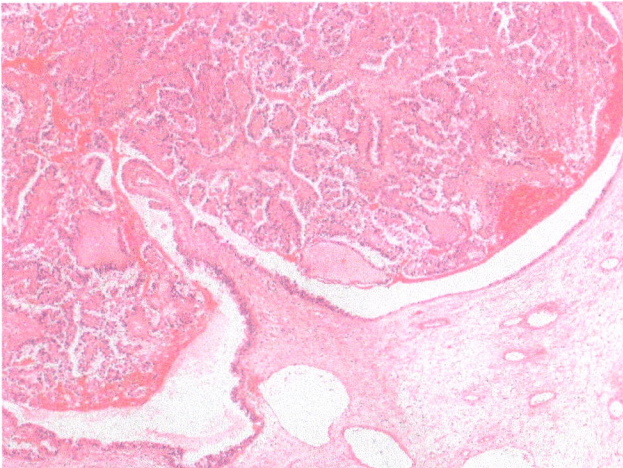

Figure 1. Clear cell carcinoma of the ovary arising in the lumen of an endometrioma, lined by columnar endometrioid cells. Hematoxylin and eosin × 150.

All patients underwent surgery, received chemotherapy and were followed up at our institution. Surgical staging was performed according to FIGO guidelines for ovarian cancer, including total abdominal hysterectomy, bilateral salpingo-oophorectomy, omentectomy and the removal of all macroscopic diseases [26]. All pathological analysis was performed by the same gynecologic pathologist.

The patients were divided into two groups according to histology (EAEOC or ECC). Data including age at diagnosis, clinical presentation, history, disease status and pathological information, such as histology, stage, laterality, presence of concurrent endometrial carcinoma and macroscopic appearance of the tumor at surgery, were collected from surgical and pathology reports. The macroscopic appearance of the tumor was reported as the rate between the solid and cystic components at gross histology, expressed as a percentage. Stages higher than IIA were classified as advanced, while lower stages were considered early. The history of endometriosis, accounting for either previous surgery for endometriosis, or the ultrasound detection of an endometriotic cyst, was indicated. All the above-mentioned variables were described for each of the two groups and statistically compared. Statistical analyses were performed using Statistical Package for Social Science (SPSS) version 28.0 (SPSS Inc., Chicago, IL, USA) and the R environment. The Pearson chi-square test or the Student's t-test were used to assess the significance of differences in clinical and pathological variables between the two groups. We also investigated the difference in FIGO stage across time points between ECC and EAEOC by means of the regression model "stage $= (\alpha_{0\ EAEOC} + I_{ECC}\ \alpha_0) + (\alpha_{1\ EAEOC} + I_{ECC}\ \alpha_1)\ time$" where "$\alpha_{0\ EAEOC}$" and "$\alpha_{1\ EAEOC}$" are the intercept and the slope of the model for EAEOC patients, respectively; "I_{ECC}" is the dummy variable for ECC patients and "α_0" and "α_1" are the intercepts difference and the slopes difference between EAEOC and ECC patients, respectively. In all analyses, a p value of <0.05 was considered statistically significant.

3. Results

Medical records and pathologic specimens were available for $n = 48$ patients diagnosed with endometriosis-associated ovarian cancer in the considered time interval. Of these, $n = 26$ (54%) had EAEOC and $n = 22$ (46%) had ECC. The clinical and morphological characteristics of the two groups are shown in Table 1. Age was not significantly different between the two groups. Interestingly, seven patients in the ECC group (32%) were previously diagnosed or operated on for endometriosis, while only one patient (4%) in the EAEOC group reported a history of endometriosis ($p = 0.01$). Considering the clinical presentation, the symptoms did not differ statistically between the two groups, except for abdominal pain, which was significantly more frequent in the EAEOC group (46% vs. 14%, $p = 0.02$) (Table 1).

As shown in Table 1, 85% of EAEOC subjects were diagnosed with early-stage disease, in contrast to 59% of the ECC subjects, as the FIGO stages were significantly different between the two groups ($p = 0.04$). The incidence of bilaterality was significantly higher in the EAOEC group as compared to the ECC group (35% vs. 5%, $p = 0.01$). Additionally, considering the macroscopic appearance of the tumor, the solid/cystic rate at histological examination was significantly higher for the EAOEC group (57.7 ± 7.9% vs. 30.9 ± 7.5%, $p = 0.02$). Interestingly, 10 patients in the EAEOC group (38%) had a diagnosis of synchronous endometrial cancer while none of the patients in the ECC group did ($p = 0.001$).

Trends in FIGO stage at diagnosis, as a function of the year of detection, are reported in Figure 2 in relation to the specific histotype. According to the multivariate regression analysis, the year of diagnosis was a significant predictor of FIGO stage for the clear cell histotype ($p = 0.02$) while it was not for the EAEOC histotype ($p = 0.32$; slopes difference: $p = 0.02$).

Table 1. Clinical and pathological characteristics of endometriosis-associated ovarian tumors.

Characteristics	EAEOC (n = 26)	ECC (n = 22)	p
Age (mean ± SD)	53.4 ± 9.1	53.1 ± 10.1	0.9
Symptoms			
Abdominal pain	12 (46%)	3 (14%)	**0.02**
Abdominal distension	11 (42%)	5 (23%)	0.13
Vaginal bleeding	7 (27%)	2 (9%)	0.11
Fatigue	1 (4%)	1 (5%)	0.70
Incidental diagnosis	6 (23%)	4 (18%)	0.54
Ascites	3 (11%)	0	0.15
History of endometriosis	1 (4%)	7 (32%)	**0.01**
FIGO stage			**0.04**
Early stage	22 (85%)	13 (59%)	
Advanced stage	4 (15%)	9 (41%)	
Grading			**<0.001**
1	10 (40%)	0	
2	8 (30%)	0	
3	8 (30%)	22 (100%)	
Tumor side			**0.01**
Monolateral	17 (65%)	21 (95%)	
Bilateral involvement	9 (35%)	1 (5%)	
Solid/cystic tumor rate (%)	57.7 ± 7.9	30.9 ± 7.5	**0.02**
Synchronous endometrial cancer	10	0	**0.001**

Bold: Means statistically significant ($p < 0.05$).

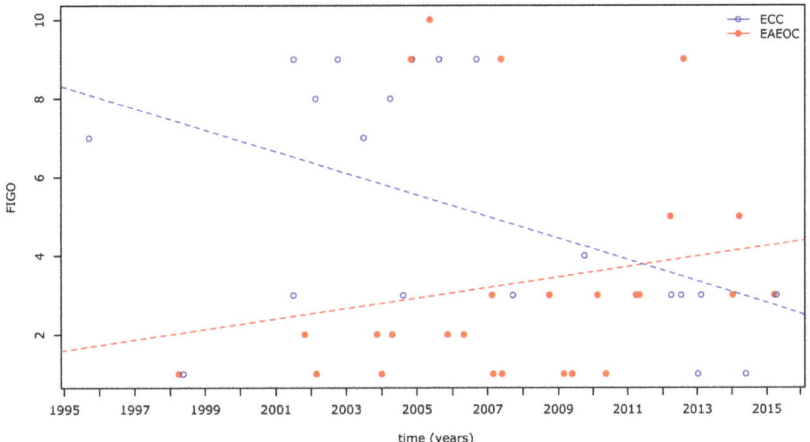

Figure 2. Trends of FIGO stage at diagnosis according to the year of detection for EAEOC and ECC.

4. Discussion

The malignant transformation of endometriosis is, in general, a rare event that occurs in between 0.7–1.6% of women [27].

In a recent systematic review and meta-analysis by Kvaskoff and collaborators, it has been estimated that endometriosis is associated with a greater risk of clear cell and endometrioid histotypes, equal to 3.4-fold and 2.3-fold, respectively [9]. In particular, these authors pooled the results of 24 studies (case–control and cohort studies), published between January 1990 and January 2020, on the relationship between endometriosis and ovarian cancer, and investigat the impact of endometriosis on the risk and prognosis of ovarian cancer (summary relative risk—[SRR] = 1.93, 95% confidential interval—[CI] = 1.68–2.22). A stronger association with endometriosis was found for the clear cell histotype (SRR = 3.44,

95% CI = 2.82–4.20) while a still significant but weaker association was reported for the endometrioid histotype (SRR = 2.33, 95% CI = 1.82–2.98) [9].

The carcinogenic pathways underlying the malignant transformation of endometriosis are not completely clear. Endometriosis-associated ovarian carcinogenesis is a multistep process, in which a precursor lesion, such as atypical endometriosis, harboring key mutations, progressively accumulates genetic and epigenetic changes, which are promoted by the inflammatory, hyperestrogenic environment and oxidative milieu of the endometriotic lesion [2].

In particular, it has been proposed that the transition from endometrioma to atypical endometriosis may be caused by oxidative stress, due to reactive oxygen species developing within the blood, which are present in endometriomas. This causes genetic mutations, initially affecting the oncosuppressor gene *ARID1A* and subsequently affecting *PIK3CA*. The accumulation of these genetic alterations induces the transition from atypical endometriosis to ovarian cancer [2].

There is, however, an increasing body of evidence from clinicopathological studies suggesting that separate pathways of malignant degeneration of endometriosis might be involved in clear cell and endometrioid tumors and that their relationship with endometriosis might be different [19]. In particular, atypical endometriosis, meaning cytological and histological atypia such as a hyperchromatic nucleus, an increased nucleus-cytoplasm ratio and cell crowding, is considered to be a direct precursor of epithelial ovarian cancer. In fact, it is present in 60–80% of tumors associated with endometriosis, but it is more frequently associated with clear cells tumors (36%), compared with endometrioid cancer (23%) [4]. Furthermore, the trigger of carcinogenesis in clear cell carcinomas may be due to oxidative stress generated by iron-related substances, due to the repeated hemorrhages that occur in endometriosis, while for endometrioid cancer, Müllerian metaplasia has been considered to be the main mechanism involved [4].

From a biological standpoint, support for this hypothesis derives from the investigation of the hepatocyte nuclear factor (HNF-1β) overexpression in clear cell carcinoma of the ovary associated with endometriosis. In fact, from an immunohistochemical point of view, this factor is only detected in eutopic and ectopic endometrium and in clear-cell-type tumors. This supports the theory of endometriosis expressing HNF-1β as the precursor of endometriosis-associated clear cell carcinoma [20]. Conversely, the absence of HNF-1β expression in endometrioid histology and in ovarian cortical inclusion cysts would support the metaplastic transformation of the inclusion cysts into a Müllerian epithelium as a precursor of endometrioid tumor development [20]. In addition, ovarian cancer associated with endometriosis is correlated with the same molecular features that are present in endometriosis (particularly in the atypical variant) and type 1 ovarian cancer, such as PIK3CA and *KRAS* activating mutations and *ARID1A* and *PTEN* inactivating mutations, although there are differences in the frequency of these alterations between the two subtypes of ovarian cancer. *ARID1A* mutations are found in 46% of ECC and 30% of EAEOC, PIK3CA mutations are present in 41–57% of ECC and in 30–48% of EAEOC and finally, PTEN is mutated in 25% of ECC and in 20% of EAEOC. Moreover, *KRAS* and *CTNNB1* are mutated in 29% and 40% of EAEOC, respectively, and in 7% and 3% of ECC, respectively [6,27]. From a clinical standpoint, very few studies have highlighted the different behavior of these two histotypes with respect to endometriosis.

Indeed, we agree on the existence of a dichotomy in the etiology of the two different ovarian tumors correlated with endometriosis. However, evidence from our previous studies and the common molecular alterations found to be shared between endometriosis-associated endometrioid ovarian cancer and type I endometrial carcinoma has led us to postulate some different novel hypotheses, suggesting a parallelism between endometrial and ovarian endometrioid tumors [24,25]. It is known that the association between endometrial neoplasm and ovarian endometrioid cancer occurs in 3.1–10.0% of patients with endometrial cancer and in 10% of those with ovarian cancer [28]. In fact, in a recent retrospective cohort study by Ishizaka and colleagues has demonstrated that endometrial cancer associated with endometriosis has a high probability of being simultaneous at ovarian carcinoma, in particular, endometrioid histotype is the most common histological subtype present [29]. Moreover, different types of gene-based biomarkers such as *ARID1A*, *PIK3CA*, *KRAS* and *CTNNB1* are recurrently mutated in endometrial cancer type I, endometriosis and endometriosis-associated ovarian tumors [30]. According to this idea, which is summarized in Figure 3, the original precursor of EAEOC might be found in the endometrium, where an already mutated endometrial cell might lead, via retrograde menstruation, to the development of ovarian endometriosis.

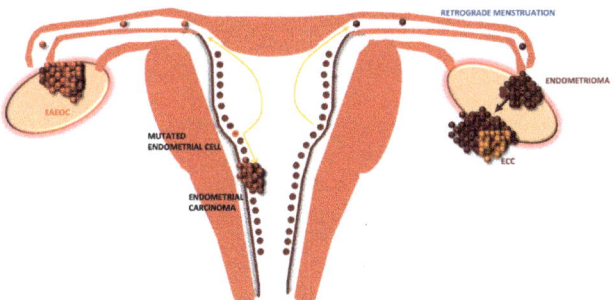

Figure 3. Dichotomy in the histogenesis of endometriosis-associated ovarian cancer histotypes. In EAEOC, the original precursor might derive from the endometrium, while evidence would support ECC carcinogenesis to occur within the endometrioma. EAEOC: endometriosis-associated endometrioid ovarian carcinoma; ECC: endometriosis-associated clear cell ovarian carcinoma.

Interestingly, in the current series, we confirmed the detection of synchronous endometrial carcinoma only in EAEOC and not in ECC. Conversely, the endometriotic cyst, which is often detected several years before, might be the setting for the development of clear cell carcinomas, but not for endometrioid ovarian cancer. In fact, the carcinogenesis underlying the transformation of endometriosis to clear cell carcinoma would be different: it might originate from and slowly progress within the endometriotic cyst, due to the effect of oxidative stress and inflammation, which involves different pathways [2,3,6]. This hypothesis for a dichotomy in the etiology of the two histotypes finds further support in the current analysis. Firstly, a history of known endometriosis was reported more frequently in the ECC group than the EAEOC group, with a statistically significant difference. Moreover, the cystic nature of clear cell carcinoma might be explained by the significantly higher detection of a unilateral lesion in the ECC group, considering that endometriomas are rarely bilateral. In line with this observation, the solid/cystic rate in the ECC group at macroscopic histology was significantly lower than the EAEOC group. Arguments against the theory by Kajihara et al. include (i) the demonstration by various authors of the endometrioid histology in synchronous ovarian and endometrial carcinomas associated with endometriosis which is not consistent with the endometrioid tumor development from the Müllerian epithelium [29,30]; (ii) evidence supporting different origins for the various forms of endometriosis [8] does not tend to indicate two different histogeneses for the endometriotic cyst, as the theory of Kajihara and coworkers would imply. Endometriosis in different sites might indeed have a different histogenesis. On the other hand, the possibility that clear cell carcinoma cancer might originate from pre-existing endometriosis, derived from regurgitated endometrial cells on the ovarian surface, contrasts with the observation that in 61% of ovarian carcinomas, which develop secondary to pre-existing, benign-appearing endometriomas which have a long latency interval (mean 4.5 years) between the benign and the malign entities, the histologic findings are clear cell carcinoma [27,31].

It is important to consider that if the theory of slow development of clear cell carcinoma within an already known endometrioma is true, then we would expect ultrasound monitoring to be effective only in the early detection of ECC, but not EAEOC. As a matter of fact, in our study population, between 1995 and 2016, a significantly decreasing trend in the FIGO stage at diagnosis was identified for ECC, but not for EAEOC, and the difference between the trends was statistically significant ($p = 0.02$). This could find a possible explanation in the diffusion of ultrasound as a follow-up technology for ovarian endometriotic cysts and in the effort of some authors to study and describe the peculiar and early sonographic appearance of the malignant degeneration of endometriomas [7,32,33].

In particular, from an ultrasonographic standpoint, endometriosis-associated endometrioid carcinomas are mainly unilateral, unilocular-solid and often contain papillary projections. Conversely, the typical ultrasound pattern of endometrioid ovarian carcinomas not developing from endometriosis is cockade-like, which refers to a cyst with a large central solid component entrapped within locules [32]. Clear cell tumors do not show a typical pattern, as this type of tumor more often shows a ground-glass echogenicity of cyst fluid [33].

The clinical implications of this finding are important considering that clear cell carcinoma is known for its low chemosensitivity and poor prognosis in advanced-stage disease, while the survival rate of adequately staged IA disease is greater than 95% [34,35]. The stage at diagnosis of clear cell carcinomas arising from endometriosis is expected to further decrease with the increasing use of ultrasound in the follow-up of endometriotic cysts, thus allowing clinicians to identify a subset of patients with a better prognosis. Moreover, a meta-analysis by Chen and colleagues highlighted better overall survival (OS) and progression-free survival (PSF) in patients with endometriosis-associated ovarian cancer compared to women with neoplasms not related to endometriosis [10]. More studies are needed to understand if there is a difference in terms of OS and PSF between clear cell carcinoma and endometrioid carcinoma associated with endometriosis.

Our study has several limitations, with the main limitation being its small sample size; these results should be interpreted with caution and need to be confirmed in larger cohorts. The next step of this study could involve the separate investigation of clear cell and endometrioid ovarian tumors with and without associated endometriosis. This more complete design and the simultaneous increase in the number of cases will be helpful in better defining the differences in terms of clinical behavior, outcomes and prognosis between these two different entities. Another limitation is the lack of molecular characterization of these tumors, which could be helpful in understanding the biology underlying carcinogenesis and its relationship with endometriosis.

5. Conclusions

Among endometriosis-associated ovarian cancers, ECC, unlike EAEOC, seems to be characterized by slow development within an endometriotic cyst, thus representing a subset of diseases where ultrasound could be effective in the early detection of malignant degeneration. However, even if the clinical evidence suggests that there is a dichotomy in the etiology of endometriosis-associated ovarian cancer, the biology underlying carcinogenesis still remains unclear and this should therefore be addressed by further larger studies.

Author Contributions: Conceptualization, A.B. and G.M.; methodology, A.B.; software, A.B.; validation, A.B., G.M., A.A., G.T., E.R., L.B., G.C., G.C., R.C., F.P., G.S., C.S. and M.C.; formal analysis, A.B. and A.A.; investigation, A.B.; resources, A.B., L.B., E.R., G.C., F.P. and R.C.; data curation, A.B. and G.S.; writing—original draft preparation, A.B.; writing—review and editing, A.B., G.S.; visualization G.S.; supervision, A.B., G.M. and M.C.; project administration, A.B.; funding acquisition, none. All authors have read and agreed to the published version of the manuscript.

Funding: This research received no external funding.

Institutional Review Board Statement: The study was conducted in accordance with the Declaration of Helsinki and approved by the Institutional Review Board of San Raffaele Scientific Institute.

Informed Consent Statement: Informed consent was obtained from all subjects involved in the study.

Data Availability Statement: Data are stored at the Obstetrics and Gynecology Unit, San Raffaele Hospital, Milan, Italy.

Conflicts of Interest: The authors declare no conflict of interest.

References

1. Zondervan, K.T.; Becker, C.M.; Missmer, S.A. Endometriosis. *N. Engl. J. Med.* **2020**, *382*, 1244–1256. [CrossRef] [PubMed]
2. Bartiromo, L.; Schimberni, M.; Villanacci, R.; Mangili, G.; Ferrari, S.; Ottolina, J.; Salmeri, N.; Dolci, C.; Tandoi, I.; Candiani, M. A Systematic Review of Atypical Endometriosis-Associated Biomarkers. *Int. J. Mol. Sci.* **2022**, *23*, 4425. [CrossRef] [PubMed]
3. Hsiao, K.Y.; Wu, M.H.; Tsai, S.J. Epigenetic regulation of the pathological process in endometriosis. *Reprod. Med. Biol.* **2017**, *16*, 314–319. [CrossRef] [PubMed]
4. Kajiyama, H.; Suzuki, S.; Yoshihara, M.; Tamauchi, S.; Yoshikawa, N.; Niimi, K.; Shibata, K.; Kikkawa, F. Endometriosis and cancer. *Free Radic. Biol. Med.* **2019**, *133*, 186–192. [CrossRef] [PubMed]
5. França, P.R.d.C.; Lontra, A.C.P.; Fernandes, P.D. Endometriosis: A Disease with Few Direct Treatment Options. *Molecules* **2022**, *27*, 4034. [CrossRef]
6. Gaia-Oltean, A.I.; Braicu, C.; Gulei, D.; Ciortea, R.; Mihu, D.; Roman, H.; Irimie, A.; Berindan-Neagoe, I. Ovarian endometriosis, a precursor of ovarian cancer: Histological aspects, gene expression and microRNA alterations (Review). *Exp. Ther. Med.* **2021**, *21*, 243. [CrossRef]
7. Exacoustos, C.; Zupi, E.; Piccione, E. Ultrasound Imaging for Ovarian and Deep Infiltrating Endometriosis. *Semin. Reprod. Med.* **2017**, *35*, 5–24. [CrossRef]
8. Horne, A.W.; Missmer, S.A. Pathophysiology, diagnosis, and management of endometriosis. *BMJ* **2022**, *379*, e070750. [CrossRef]
9. Kvaskoff, M.; Mahamat-Saleh, Y.; Farland, L.V.; Shigesi, N.; Terry, K.L.; Harris, H.R.; Roman, H.; Becker, C.M.; As-Sanie, S.; Zondervan, K.T.; et al. Endometriosis and cancer: A systematic review and meta-analysis. *Hum. Reprod. Update* **2021**, *27*, 393–420. [CrossRef]
10. Chen, P.; Zhang, C.Y. Association Between Endometriosis and Prognosis of Ovarian Cancer: An Updated Meta-Analysis. *Front. Oncol.* **2022**, *12*, 732322. [CrossRef]
11. Shafrir, A.L.; Farland, L.V.; Shah, D.K.; Harris, H.; Kvaskoff, M.; Zondervan, K.; Missmer, S. Risk for and consequences of endometriosis: A critical epidemiologic review. *Best Pract. Res. Clin. Obstet. Gynaecol.* **2018**, *51*, 1–15. [CrossRef]
12. Vercellini, P.; Viganò, P.; Somigliana, E.; Fedele, L. Endometriosis: Pathogenesis and treatment. *Nat. Rev. Endocrinol.* **2014**, *10*, 261–275. [CrossRef]
13. Sanchez, A.M.; Viganò, P.; Somigliana, E.; Cioffi, R.; Panina-Bordignon, P.; Candiani, M. The endometriotic tissue lining the internal surface of endometrioma: Hormonal, genetic, epigenetic status, and gene expression profile. *Reprod. Sci.* **2015**, *22*, 391–401. [CrossRef]
14. Sanchez, A.M.; Viganò, P.; Somigliana, E.; Panina-Bordignon, P.; Vercellini, P.P.; Candiani, M. The distinguishing cellular and molecular features of the endometriotic ovarian cyst: From pathophysiology to the potential endometrioma-mediated damage to the ovary. *Hum. Reprod. Update* **2014**, *20*, 217–230. [CrossRef]
15. Sambasivan, S. Epithelial ovarian cancer: Review article. *Cancer Treat. Res. Commun.* **2022**, *33*, 100629. [CrossRef]
16. Köbel, M.; Kang, E.Y. The Evolution of Ovarian Carcinoma Subclassification. *Cancers* **2022**, *14*, 416. [CrossRef]
17. Rojas, V.; Hirshfield, K.M.; Ganesan, S.; Rodriguez-Rodriguez, L. Molecular Characterization of Epithelial Ovarian Cancer: Implications for Diagnosis and Treatment. *Int. J. Mol. Sci.* **2016**, *17*, 2113. [CrossRef]
18. Sarría-Santamera, A.; Khamitova, Z.; Gusmanov, A.; Terzic, M.; Polo-Santos, M.; Ortega, M.A.; Asúnsolo, A. History of Endometriosis Is Independently Associated with an Increased Risk of Ovarian Cancer. *J. Pers. Med.* **2022**, *12*, 1337. [CrossRef]
19. Mortlock, S.; Corona, R.I.; Kho, P.F.; Pharoah, P.; Seo, J.-H.; Freedman, M.L.; Gayther, S.A.; Siedhoff, M.T.; Rogers, P.A.; Leuchter, R.; et al. A multi-level investigation of the genetic relationship between endometriosis and ovarian cancer histotypes. *Cell Rep. Med.* **2022**, *3*, 100542. [CrossRef]
20. Kajihara, H.; Yamada, Y.; Shigetomi, H.; Higashiura, Y.; Kobayashi, H. The dichotomy in the histogenesis of endometriosis-associated ovarian cancer: Clear cell-type versus endometrioid-type adenocarcinoma. *Int. J. Gynecol. Pathol.* **2012**, *31*, 304–312. [CrossRef]
21. Sampson, J. Endometrial carcinoma of the ovary arising in endometrial tissue in that organ. *Arch. Surg.* **1925**, *10*, 1–72. [CrossRef]
22. Scott, R. Malignant change in endometriosis. *Obstet. Gynecol.* **1953**, *2*, 293–299.
23. Fadare, O.; Parkash, V. Pathology of Endometrioid and Clear Cell Carcinoma of the Ovary. *Surg. Pathol. Clin.* **2019**, *12*, 529–564. [CrossRef] [PubMed]
24. Mangili, G.; Bergamini, A.; Taccagni, G.; Gentile, C.; Panina, P.; Vigano, P.; Candiani, M. Unravelling the two entities of endometrioid ovarian cancer: A single center clinical experience. *Gynecol. Oncol.* **2012**, *126*, 403–407. [CrossRef] [PubMed]
25. Scarfone, G.; Bergamini, A.; Noli, S.; Villa, A.; Cipriani, S.; Taccagni, G.; Vigano, P.; Candiani, M.; Parazzini, F.; Mangili, G. Characteristics of clear cell ovarian cancer arising from endometriosis: A two center cohort study. *Gynecol. Oncol.* **2014**, *133*, 480–484. [CrossRef]
26. O'Shea, A.S. Clinical Staging of Ovarian Cancer. *Methods Mol. Biol.* **2022**, *2424*, 3–10. [CrossRef]

27. Brilhante, A.V.; Augusto, K.L.; Portela, M.C.; Sucupira, L.C.G.; Oliveira, L.A.F.; Pouchaim, A.J.; Nóbrega, L.R.M.; de Magalhães, T.F.; Sobreira, L.R.P. Endometriosis and Ovarian Cancer: An Integrative Review (Endometriosis and Ovarian Cancer). *Asian Pac. J. Cancer Prev.* **2017**, *18*, 11–16. [CrossRef]
28. Yoneoka, Y.; Yoshida, H.; Ishikawa, M.; Shimizu, H.; Uehara, T.; Murakami, T.; Kato, T. Prognostic factors of synchronous endometrial and ovarian endometrioid carcinoma. *J. Gynecol. Oncol.* **2019**, *30*, e7. [CrossRef]
29. Ishizaka, A.; Taguchi, A.; Tsuruga, T.; Maruyama, M.; Kawata, A.; Miyamoto, Y.; Tanikawa, M.; Ikemura, M.; Sone, K.; Mori, M.; et al. Endometrial cancer with concomitant endometriosis is highly associated with ovarian endometrioid carcinoma: A retrospective cohort study. *BMC Women's Health* **2022**, *22*, 332. [CrossRef]
30. Terzic, M.; Aimagambetova, G.; Kunz, J.; Bapayeva, G.; Aitbayeva, B.; Terzic, S.; Laganà, A.S. Molecular Basis of Endometriosis and Endometrial Cancer: Current Knowledge and Future Perspectives. *Int. J. Mol. Sci.* **2021**, *22*, 9274. [CrossRef]
31. Kawaguchi, R.; Tsuji, Y.; Haruta, S.; Kanayama, S.; Sakata, M.; Yamada, Y.; Fujita, H.; Saito, H.; Tsuneto, K.; Kobayashi, H. Clinicopathologic features of ovarian cancer in patients with ovarian endometrioma. *J. Obstet. Gynaecol. Res.* **2008**, *34*, 872–877. [CrossRef]
32. Moro, F.; Magoga, G.; Pasciuto, T.; Mascilini, F.; Moruzzi, M.C.; Fischerova, D.; Savelli, L.; Giunchi, S.; Mancari, R.; Franchi, D.; et al. Imaging in gynecological disease (13): Clinical and ultrasound characteristics of endometrioid ovarian cancer. *Ultrasound Obstet. Gynecol.* **2018**, *52*, 535–543. [CrossRef]
33. Pozzati, F.; Moro, F.; Pasciuto, T.; Gallo, C.; Ciccarone, F.; Franchi, D.; Mancari, R.; Giunchi, S.; Timmerman, D.; Landolfo, C.; et al. Imaging in gynecological disease (14): Clinical and ultrasound characteristics of ovarian clear cell carcinoma. *Ultrasound Obstet. Gynecol.* **2018**, *52*, 792–800. [CrossRef]
34. Gadducci, A.; Multinu, F.; Cosio, S.; Carinelli, S.; Ghioni, M.; Aletti, G.D. Clear cell carcinoma of the ovary: Epidemiology, pathological and biological features, treatment options and clinical outcomes. *Gynecol Oncol.* **2021**, *162*, 741–750. [CrossRef]
35. Ceppi, L.; Grassi, T.; Galli, F.; Buda, A.; Aletti, G.; Lissoni, A.A.; Adorni, M.; Garbi, A.; Colombo, N.; Bonazzi, C.; et al. Early-stage clear cell ovarian cancer compared to high-grade histological subtypes: An outcome exploratory analysis in two oncology centers. *Gynecol. Oncol.* **2021**, *160*, 64–70. [CrossRef]

Disclaimer/Publisher's Note: The statements, opinions and data contained in all publications are solely those of the individual author(s) and contributor(s) and not of MDPI and/or the editor(s). MDPI and/or the editor(s) disclaim responsibility for any injury to people or property resulting from any ideas, methods, instructions or products referred to in the content.

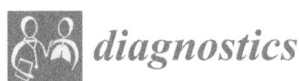

Article

Endometrioid Carcinomas of the Ovaries and Endometrium Involving Endocervical Polyps: Comprehensive Clinicopathological Analyses

Jihee Sohn, Yurimi Lee * and Hyun-Soo Kim *

Department of Pathology and Translational Genomics, Samsung Medical Center, Sungkyunkwan University School of Medicine, Seoul 06351, Korea
* Correspondence: yrm.lee@samsung.com (Y.L.); hyun-soo.kim@samsung.com (H.-S.K.)

Abstract: While synchronous ovarian and endometrial endometrioid carcinomas (ECs) have long been described in the literature, ovarian or endometrial EC involving concomitant endocervical polyp (ECP) has not yet been reported. This study aimed to investigate the histological types and prevalence of gynecological tumors co-existing with ECP and to comprehensively analyze the clinicopathological characteristics of ovarian and endometrial ECs involving ECPs. We searched for ECP cases associated with premalignant lesions or malignancies of the female genital tract occurring between March 2019 and February 2022. We then investigated the histological types and prevalence of gynecological tumors co-existing with ECP. In addition, we reviewed electronic medical records and pathology slides to collect the clinicopathological features of four patients with ovarian or endometrial EC involving ECP. We found 429 ECPs over the three-year study period. Of these, 68 (15.9%) were associated with premalignant or malignant lesions occurring in the uterine cervix, endometrium, and ovaries. Four of these cases, including two (0.5%) ovarian grade 3 ECs and two (0.5%) endometrial grade 1 ECs, involved ECPs. In the former cases (cases 1 and 2), ECs involving ECPs exhibited similar morphology and immunohistochemical staining results to those of advanced-stage ovarian EC. In the latter cases (cases 3 and 4), the histological and immunophenotypical features of EC involving ECP were identical to those of primary endometrial EC, despite the lack of tumor involvement in the myometrium, lower uterine segment, and cervical stroma as well as the absence of lymphovascular invasion and lymph node metastasis. In all cases, no evidence of benign endometriosis, endometrial hyperplasia without atypia, or atypical hyperplasia/endometrial intraepithelial neoplasm within ECP or the adjacent endocervical tissue was noted. Considering our results, the involvement of ECP by EC may have been caused by an implantation metastasis from the ovarian (cases 1 and 2) or endometrial (cases 3 and 4) EC. To the best of our knowledge, this is the first exploration of the synchronous occurrence of endometrial or ovarian EC and ECP involvement. Implantation metastasis via transtubal and trans-endometrial cavity migration may have been the pathogenic mechanism of ECP involvement.

Keywords: cervix; endocervical polyp; ovary; endometrium; endometrioid carcinoma; implantation metastasis

Citation: Sohn, J.; Lee, Y.; Kim, H.-S. Endometrioid Carcinomas of the Ovaries and Endometrium Involving Endocervical Polyps: Comprehensive Clinicopathological Analyses. Diagnostics 2022, 12, 2339. https://doi.org/10.3390/diagnostics12102339

Academic Editors: Cinzia Giacometti and Kathrin Ludwig

Received: 31 August 2022
Accepted: 21 September 2022
Published: 27 September 2022

Publisher's Note: MDPI stays neutral with regard to jurisdictional claims in published maps and institutional affiliations.

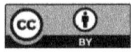

Copyright: © 2022 by the authors. Licensee MDPI, Basel, Switzerland. This article is an open access article distributed under the terms and conditions of the Creative Commons Attribution (CC BY) license (https://creativecommons.org/licenses/by/4.0/).

1. Introduction

Endocervical polyps (ECPs) are benign proliferative lesions of the uterine cervix that typically occur in the endocervical canal [1]. Stromal overgrowth and reactive epithelial hyperplasia associated with repeated episodes of inflammation, an abnormal local response to increased estrogen levels, and the local congestion of cervical stromal blood vessels are involved in the development of ECP [1,2]. More than half of the patients with ECP are asymptomatic, with the ECPs being discovered incidentally during routine gynecological examinations. However, symptomatic ECPs manifest as vaginal discharge, leukorrhea, menorrhagia, metrorrhagia, postcoital bleeding, and postmenopausal bleeding [2].

Endometrioid carcinoma (EC) of the endometrium is the most common histological type of endometrial carcinoma. The microscopic appearance of this tumor resembles that of a normal proliferative-phase endometrium, with variable degrees of glandular complexity and nuclear pleomorphism [3]. The diagnosis of endometrial EC is usually based on clinical findings and imaging and confirmed with endometrial curettage. In addition, EC of the ovaries accounts for 15% of epithelial ovarian carcinomas [4] and is associated with endometriosis in most cases [5,6]. Ovarian EC, morphologically similar to endometrial EC, is characterized by a confluent back-to-back arrangement of variable-sized glands lined by pseudostratified columnar epithelium with elongated nuclei [7–9].

Primary EC of the uterine cervix has often been misclassified in the literature due to the lack of clear-cut diagnostic criteria [10]. Based on a new classification system, the International Endocervical Adenocarcinoma Criteria and Classification [11–13], cervical EC is a rare histological type of human papillomavirus (HPV)-independent endocervical adenocarcinoma (EAC), with an overall prevalence of 1.1% [13]. Determining whether EC has occurred in the uterine corpus or the cervix is difficult, but this distinction is important as the optimal management of EC and EAC differs significantly.

Synchronous endometrial and ovarian ECs have long been described in the literature. However, the synchronous occurrence of either endometrial or ovarian EC and ECP involvement has not yet been reported. This phenomenon poses diagnostic challenges, as determining whether they are independent primary tumors or metastases of each other, as well as what the original tumor may be, is difficult [14]. Clinical presentation, previous gynecological history, and ancillary tests, such as immunohistochemical staining, are helpful in correctly diagnosing morphologically challenging cases. An accurate pathological diagnosis is fundamental for proper clinical practices and optimal patient outcomes.

We recently encountered four cases of ovarian or endometrial EC involving ECP. The reported prevalence of malignancies involving ECPs is 0.1–0.5% [1], and a thorough literature review revealed no information about EC involving ECP. In this study, we investigated the histological types and prevalence of gynecological tumors co-existing with ECP. We then comprehensively analyzed the pathological characteristics of four patients with ovarian or endometrial EC involving ECP and discussed their clinical significance and the possible pathogenesis. Our observations may encourage pathologists to recognize and accurately diagnose this rare but distinct occurrence.

2. Materials and Methods

2.1. Case Selection

We searched in the departmental archives for cases matching the keywords "endocervical polyp" and "cervical polyp" occurring between March 2019 and February 2022. A total of 429 cases of ECP were included in this study, of which 68 (15.9%) were ECPs co-existing with premalignant lesions or malignancies arising in any site of the gynecological tract and 4 (0.9%) were microscopically identified areas of EC involving the surface and stroma of ECPs. Representative formalin-fixed, paraffin-embedded tissue blocks were used for immunohistochemical staining.

2.2. Clinical Data Collection

The following clinical information was obtained from electronic medical records and pathology reports: age of patients, presenting symptoms, previous gynecological history, preoperative imaging findings, clinical impressions, cervical punch biopsy results, history of endocervical curettage and endometrial curettage, data on neoadjuvant chemotherapy use, surgical procedures, final pathological diagnosis, International Federation of Gynecology and Obstetrics (FIGO) stages [15], data on postoperative treatment and recurrence, disease-free survival, treatments for recurrence, survival status, and overall survival.

2.3. Pathological Data Collection

Pathological information was obtained from the slide review. For ECs involving ECP, histological type and grade [16], the greatest dimension, invasion depth into the polyp stroma, endocervical glandular extension, polypectomy resection margin involvement, the presence of endometriosis, atypical hyperplasia/endometrial intraepithelial neoplasm (AH/EIN), and lymphovascular invasion (LVI) were collected. For endometrial ECs, histological type and grade [16]; the largest dimension; myometrial invasion depth; cervical stromal extension; involvement of the lower uterine segment, uterine serosa, and parametrium; lymph node metastasis; and adnexal extension were collected. For ovarian ECs, histological type and grade [16]; the largest dimension; ovarian surface extension; involvement of the salpinx, uterus, and peritoneum; lymph node metastasis; and the presence of ovarian endometriotic cyst were collected.

2.4. Immunohistochemical Staining

We performed immunohistochemical staining based on previously described methods [17–22]. Immunohistochemical staining was performed using the Bond Polymer Intense Detection System (Leica Biosystems, Buffalo Grove, IL, USA). Briefly, 4-μm-thick sections cut from formalin-fixed, paraffin-embedded tissue blocks were deparaffinized in xylene and rehydrated through a series of graded alcohols. After antigen retrieval, endogenous peroxidases were quenched with hydrogen peroxide. The sections were incubated with primary antibodies against estrogen receptor (ER, 1:150, clone 6F11, catalog number ER-6F11-L-CE, Novocastra, Leica Biosystems, Buffalo Grove, IL, USA), progesterone receptor (PR, 1:100, clone 16, catalog number PGR-312-L-CE, Novocastra, Leica Biosystems, Buffalo Grove, IL, USA), p16 (prediluted, clone E6H4, catalog number 805-4713, Ventana Medical Systems, Oro Valley, AZ, USA), p53 (1:200, clone DO-7, catalog number NCL-L-p53-DO7, Novocastra, Leica Biosystems, Buffalo Grove, IL, USA), and Wilms tumor 1 (WT1, 1:800, clone 6F-H2, catalog number 348M-98, Cell Marque, Rocklin, CA, USA). A biotin-free polymeric horseradish peroxidase-linker antibody conjugate system was used with a BOND-MAX automated immunostainer (Leica Biosystems, Buffalo Grove, IL, USA). After chromogenic visualization using 3,3′-diaminobenzidine, the sections were counterstained with hematoxylin, dehydrated in graded alcohols and xylene, and then embedded in a mounting solution. Appropriate controls were stained concurrently. Positive controls were luminal A-type invasive breast carcinoma for ER and PR; cervical high-grade squamous intraepithelial lesion (HSIL) for p16; and ovarian high-grade serous carcinoma for p53 and WT1. Negative controls were prepared by substituting non-immune serum for primary antibodies, which resulted in undetectable staining.

2.5. Immunohistochemical Interpretation

Each immunostained slide was scored by two pathologists [18,23–29]. Staining intensities of hormone receptors and WT1 were designated as either weak, moderate, or strong, and staining proportions were determined in increments of 5% across a 0–100% range and classified as negative, focal (<50%), or diffuse ($\geq$50%). Expression patterns of p16 were considered diffuse and strong positivity when p16 was expressed in the nuclei and/or cytoplasm with continuous and strong staining. All other p16 expression patterns, including focal nuclear staining, wispy, blob-like, puddled, and scattered cytoplasmic staining, were interpreted as patchy positivity [1,22,23,25,28]. Similarly, p53 expression patterns were considered aberrant when any of the following features were observed: diffuse and strong nuclear immunoreactivity in $\geq$75% of tumor cells (i.e., over-expression); no nuclear immunoreactivity in any tumor cell (i.e., complete absence); or unequivocal cytoplasmic staining (i.e., cytoplasmic pattern). Immunostained slides exhibiting a variable proportion of tumor cell nuclei expressing p53 with mild-to-moderate intensity were considered wild type [30].

3. Results

3.1. The Prevalence and Histological Types of Gynecological Tumors Co-Existing with ECP

As shown in Table 1, of the 429 patients with ECP identified, 68 (15.9%) had premalignant or malignant lesions arising in the uterine cervix, endometrium, and ovaries. Most of the cervical tumors (17/20; 85.0%) involved ECP, with HSIL being the most common (11/17; 64.7%). Additionally, three of the five patients who underwent radical hysterectomy for squamous cell carcinomas (SCCs) had ECPs, and endocervical adenocarcinoma in situ (AIS) involving ECP was present in two patients. We also found one case of stratified mucin-producing intraepithelial lesion (SMILE) co-existing with HSIL, in which ECP was involved by both SMILE and HSIL. ECPs presented as separate lesions in one patient with HSIL and AIS and two patients with SCC.

Table 1. The histological types and prevalence of gynecological tumors co-existing with ECP.

Origin	Relationship with ECP	Histological Type	Number of Cases (Prevalence)
Uterine cervix	Involving ECP	HSIL	11 (2.6%)
		SCC	3 (0.7%)
		AIS	2 (0.5%)
		SMILE and HSIL	1 (0.2%)
	Separate	SCC	2 (0.5%)
		AIS and HSIL	1 (0.2%)
EM	Involving ECP	EC	2 (0.5%)
	Separate	EC	14 (3.3%)
		AH/EIN	6 (1.4%)
		EC and CCC	1 (0.2%)
		SC	1 (0.2%)
Ovary	Involving ECP	EC	2 (0.5%)
	Separate	HGSC	14 (3.3%)
		CCC	3 (0.7%)
		EC	2 (0.5%)
		MC	2 (0.5%)
		LGSC	1 (0.2%)
Total			68 (15.9%)

AIS: Adenocarcinoma in situ; AH/EIN: atypical hyperplasia/endometrial intraepithelial neoplasm; CCC: clear cell carcinoma; EC: endometrial carcinoma; EM: endometrium; HGSC: high-grade serous carcinoma; HSIL: high-grade squamous intraepithelial lesion; LGSC: low-grade serous carcinoma; MC: mucinous carcinoma; SCC: squamous cell carcinoma; SMILE: stratified mucin-producing intraepithelial lesion.

In contrast with the cervical tumors, most of the endometrial and ovarian tumors associated with ECP did not directly involve the polyps. The most common endometrial tumor associated with ECP was EC (16/24; 66.7%), while 14 of the 16 endometrial EC cases simply co-existed with ECPs in the hysterectomy specimens, without direct involvement. Moreover, six ECP cases with endometrial AH/EIN had no direct involvement with the tumor, and 14 patients who underwent debulking surgery for ovarian high-grade serous carcinoma (HGSC) showed benign incidental ECPs in their hysterectomy specimens. Three clear cell carcinomas, two ECs, two mucinous carcinomas, and one low-grade serous carcinoma of the ovary also co-existed with ECP, without polyp or uterine cervix involvement. Therefore, two cases of endometrial EC and two cases of ovarian EC involving ECPs were ultimately detected. We investigated the clinicopathological features of four patients with ovarian or endometrial EC involving ECP.

3.2. Clinical Presentations of Four Patients with EC Involving ECP

Case 1: A 33-year-old woman with polycystic ovary syndrome was referred to our institution for the evaluation and management of adnexal masses, after visiting an outside hospital with lower abdominal discomfort. Abdominopelvic computed tomography (CT) and magnetic resonance imaging (MRI) revealed an 8.6 cm solid and cystic left ovarian mass and a 4.0 cm solid right ovarian mass (Figure 1A). An omental cake was noted, and some metastatic nodules were also identified in the cul-de-sac and right round ligament. Additionally, the retroperitoneal lymph nodes were mildly enlarged, and the endometrium was unremarkable. Following three cycles of neoadjuvant chemotherapy with paclitaxel and carboplatin, the patient underwent interval debulking surgery, including a total hysterectomy with bilateral salpingo-oophorectomy, pelvic and para-aortic lymph node dissection, omentectomy, peritoneal mass excision, and low anterior resection. The final pathological diagnosis was grade 3 EC of the bilateral ovaries, involving the omentum, rectosigmoid colon, and peritoneum (FIGO stage IIIC). We also identified a 2.4 cm polypoid mass originating from the upper endocervix, with histological examination revealing several areas of EC that spread along the surface and invaded the polyp stroma. She received three cycles of post-operative adjuvant chemotherapy with paclitaxel and carboplatin. However, she presented with chest wall pain 49 months postoperatively, and chest CT and thoracic wall MRI revealed a 2.8 cm metastatic mass involving the upper sternal body and right parasternal area. She underwent complete surgical excision. Pathological examination of the mass confirmed the metastasis of ovarian EC to the sternum and rib. She is currently alive without evidence of recurrent disease, 67 months postoperatively.

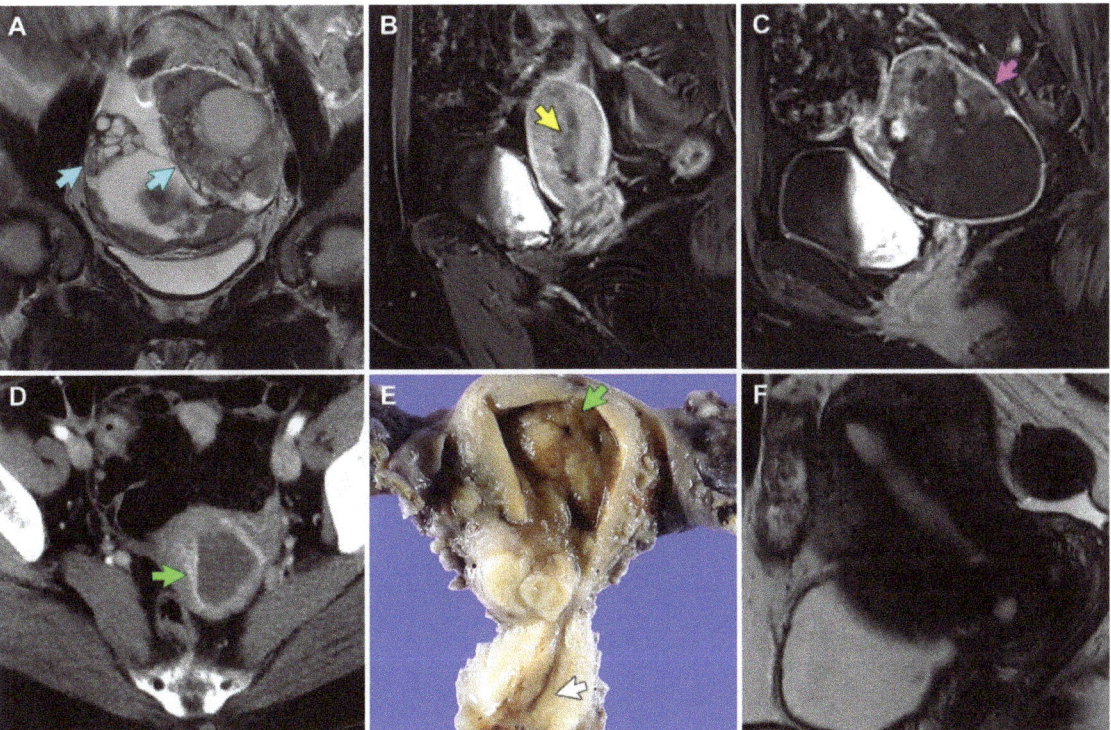

Figure 1. MRI, CT, and gross findings. (**A**) Case 1: T2-weighted coronal MR image reveals solid and cystic bilateral ovarian masses (blue arrows). (**B**,**C**) Case 2: T1-weighted Dixon sagittal MR images reveal (**B**) 3.4 cm endometrial mass (yellow arrow) and (**C**) 8.6 cm solid and cystic left ovarian mass (purple arrow). (**D**) Case 3: Contrast-enhanced CT image reveals a 1 cm endometrial mass (green arrow) and hematometra. (**E**) Case 3: An irregularly elevated mass is noted in the endometrium. The endometrial cavity is distended with blood. The endocervix (white arrow) appears unremarkable. (**F**) Case 4: T2-weighted sagittal MR image reveals no identifiable lesion in the endometrium.

Case 2: A 57-year-old woman was referred to our institution for the evaluation and management of uterine and adnexal masses, after visiting an outside hospital with lower abdominal pain and undergoing abdominopelvic CT and MRI. She had a history of hypertension, diabetes mellitus, pulmonary tuberculosis, and hypothyroidism. Imaging revealed a 3.4 cm endometrial mass with soft tissue density (Figure 1B) and an 8.6 cm solid and cystic left ovarian mass (Figure 1C). The retroperitoneal lymph nodes were enlarged, but pelvic and iliac chain lymph nodes were unremarkable. Peritoneal seeding or hematogenous metastasis were not observed. Radiological differential diagnoses included concurrent endometrial and ovarian carcinomas or endometrial carcinoma with ovarian metastasis. The endometrial curettage was diagnosed as grade 1 EC. Total hysterectomy with bilateral salpingo-oophorectomy, pelvic lymph node dissection, pelvic peritonectomy, appendectomy, and a small bowel resection were performed. Several enlarged mesenteric lymph nodes were detected intraoperatively but could not be completely resected. The final pathological diagnosis was synchronous endometrial grade 1 EC involving more than half of the myometrium (FIGO stage IB) and ovarian grade 3 EC involving the abdominopelvic peritoneum and small bowel (FIGO stage IIIC). We also identified a 2 cm ECP originating from the upper endocervix and showing a single microscopic focus of EC, involving the surface and superficial stroma of the polyp. Follow-up CT after three cycles of post-operative adjuvant chemotherapy with paclitaxel and carboplatin revealed a newly developed 5 cm necrotic mass invading the small bowel. She was switched from chemotherapy to pembrolizumab following metastatic recurrence and is currently alive with disease, three months postoperatively.

Case 3: A 57-year-old woman was referred to our institution for the evaluation and management of an incidentally detected endocervical mass. She underwent endocervical curettage at an outside hospital and was diagnosed with grade 1 EC involving ECP. Abdominopelvic CT revealed a 1 cm endometrial mass that appeared to be invading the superficial myometrium (Figure 1D). Cervical stenosis and hematometra were noted. However, no evidence of peritoneal seeding, lymph node enlargement, or distant metastasis was noted. A total hysterectomy with bilateral salpingo-oophorectomy and pelvic lymph node dissection was performed, and the specimen revealed several foci of grade 1 EC, measuring up to 0.8 cm (Figure 1E). The tumors were confined within the endometrium (FIGO stage IA). She received no further adjuvant treatment and is currently alive without evidence of recurrent disease, 24 months postoperatively.

Case 4: A 52-year-old woman without previous gynecological history received an endocervical polypectomy at an outside hospital and was referred to our institution for further evaluation and management. The polypectomy specimen was determined to be a grade 1 EC involving ECP. Abdominopelvic MRI revealed no visible neoplastic lesions in the cervix, endometrium, lymph node, and abdominopelvic peritoneum (Figure 1F). Under the clinical impression of MRI-invisible endometrial cancer, total hysterectomy with bilateral salpingo-oophorectomy was performed. The final pathological diagnosis was grade 1 EC limited to the endometrium (FIGO stage IA). She received no further adjuvant treatment and is currently alive without evidence of recurrent disease 15 months postoperatively.

Table 2 summarizes the clinicopathological characteristics. No patient received diagnostic or therapeutic procedure before the initial pathological diagnosis. Two ovarian ECs were advanced-stage tumors, while the two endometrial ECs were early stage diseases. The two patients who underwent debulking surgery for ovarian EC later developed metastatic recurrences despite post-operative chemotherapy, whereas the two patients who underwent total hysterectomies with bilateral salpingo-oophorectomies for endometrial EC received no further treatment and experienced no disease recurrence or metastasis.

Table 2. Clinicopathological characteristics of four patients with EC involving ECP.

Case No	1	2	3	4
Age	33 years	57 years	57 years	52 years
Imaging finding	8.6-cm solid and cystic bilateral ovarian masses; borderline-sized pelvic and retroperitoneal lymph nodes; peritoneal carcinomatosis	8.6-cm solid and cystic left ovarian mass; 3.4-cm EM mass; enlarged retroperitoneal lymph nodes; peritoneal carcinomatosis	1-cm EM mass; no lymph node enlargement; no peritoneal seeding	No identifiable EM lesion; no lymph node enlargement; no peritoneal seeding
Clinical impression	Ovarian cancer	Concurrent ovarian and EM cancers	EM cancer	MRI-invisible EM cancer
Neoadjuvant chemotherapy	Paclitaxel-carboplatin (three cycles)	Not received	Not received	Not received
Surgical procedure	TH, BSO, PLND, PALND, low anterior resection, omentectomy	TH, BSO, PLND, small bowel resection, appendectomy, omentectomy, peritonectomy	TH, BSO, PLND	TH, BSO
Final pathological diagnosis	Stage IIIC grade 3 EC (ovary)	Stage IIIC grade 3 EC (ovary); stage IB grade 1 EC (EM)	Stage IA grade 1 EC (EM)	Stage IA grade 1 EC (EM)
Greatest dimension of ECP	17 mm	19 mm	11 mm	16 mm
Greatest dimension of EC	6 mm	3 mm	4 mm	10 mm
Invasion depth into polyp stroma	1 mm	0.3 mm	0.3 mm	1 mm
Polypectomy resection margin involvement (safety distance)	NA	NA	Absent (5 mm)	Absent (<1 mm)
Post-operative treatment	Paclitaxel-carboplatin (three cycles)	Paclitaxel-carboplatin (three cycles)	Not received	Not received
Post-operative recurrence	Bone (sternum and rib)	Mesentery	Absent	Absent
Disease-free survival	49 months	3 months	24 months	15 months
Treatment for recurrence	Complete surgical excision	Pembrolizumab (regimen change)	Not received	Not received
Survival status	Alive	Alive	Alive	Alive
Overall survival	67 months	3 months	24 months	15 months

BSO: Bilateral salpingo-oophorectomy; EM: endometrium; MRI: magnetic resonance imaging; PALND: para-aortic lymph node dissection; PLND: pelvic lymph node dissection; TH: total hysterectomy.

3.3. Pathological Characteristics of Four ECs Involving ECP

Case 1: A 17 mm sized ECP (Figure 2A), with a long fibrovascular stalk and elongated endocervical glands, was involved by pleomorphic EC cells. The largest dimension of EC involving ECP was 6 mm, with an invasion depth of 1 mm into the polyp stroma (Figure 2B). Poorly differentiated carcinoma involving the surface and stroma of ECP displayed solid and cribriform architecture, compatible with grade 3 EC (Figure 2C). Low-power magnification of the ovarian tumor revealed a definite involvement of the ovarian surface (Figure 2D). The primary ovarian EC showed high-grade architectural and cytological atypia, which was compatible with a grade 3 EC diagnosis (Figure 2E). A few microscopic areas resembling clear cell carcinoma were also noted (Figure 2F). The sternal metastatic tumor invaded the bony trabeculae and exhibited a poorly differentiated carcinoma, of which the histological features were similar to those of ovarian EC. Immunohistochemically, patchy p16 positivity excluded the possibility of HPV-associated EAC. The expressions of ER (Figure 2H) and PR (Figure 2I) were focal but strong in the tumor cell nuclei. Solid and cribriform architecture, high-grade nuclear atypia, and a complete lack of p53 protein expression (Figure 2J) were compatible with grade 3 EC. Negative WT1 immunoreactivity (Figure 2K) excluded the possibility of high-grade serous carcinoma.

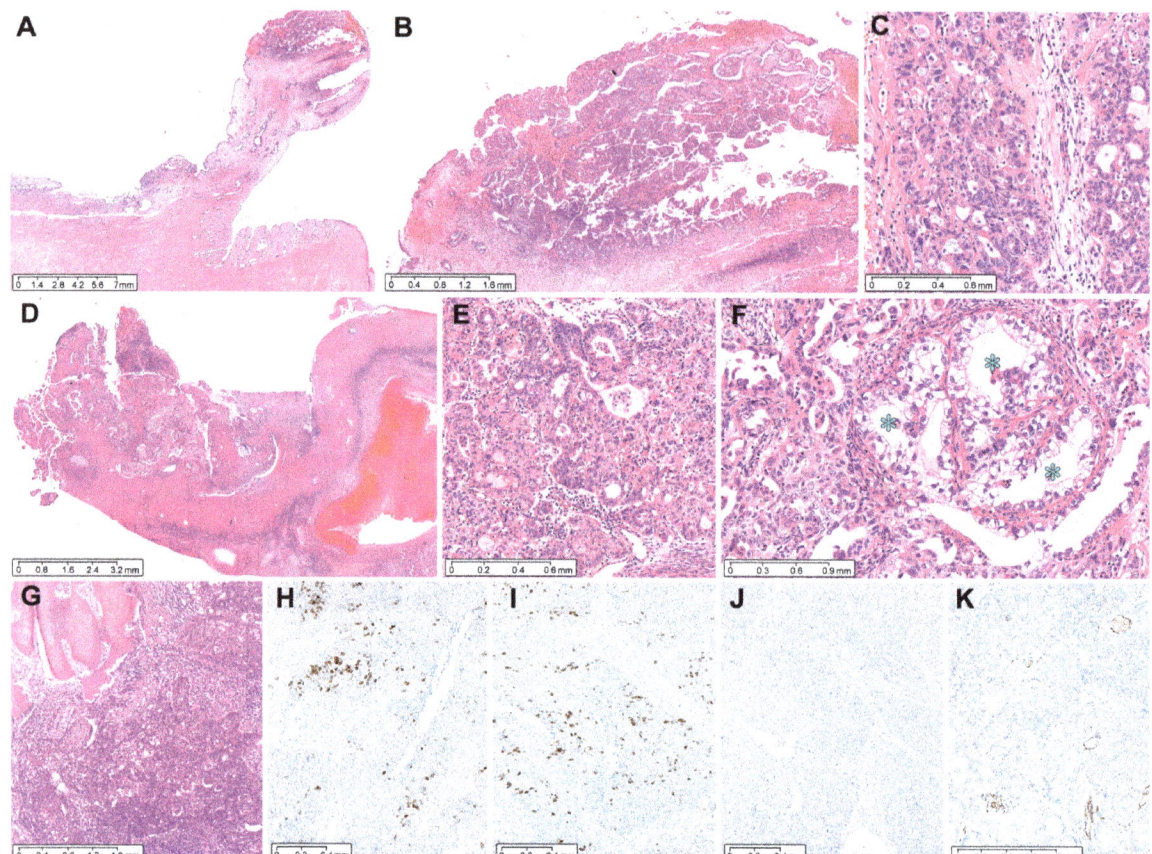

Figure 2. Grade 3 ovarian EC involving ECP: case 1. (**A**) A 1.7 cm pedunculated polyp arises from the endocervix. (**B**) Complex glandular proliferation involves the surface and stroma of ECP. The invasion depth measures 0.1 cm. (**C**) High-power magnification reveals poorly differentiated carcinoma displaying solid and cribriform architecture and high-grade cytological atypia. (**D**) The ovarian mass involves the surface and destructively invades the stroma. (**E**) The degree of cytological atypia and architecture are similar to those of poorly differentiated carcinoma involving ECP. (**F**) A few microscopic areas resembling clear cell carcinoma (blue asterisks) are noted in the ovarian tumor. (**G**) The sternal metastatic tumor invades the bony trabeculae and exhibits poorly differentiated carcinoma, and its histological features are similar to those of EC involving ECP (image (**C**)) and ovary (image (**E**)). (**H–J**) Immunohistochemical staining reveals focal and strong positivity for (**H**) estrogen receptor and (**I**) progesterone receptor and (**J**) complete absence of p53 protein expression. (**K**) Negative Wilms tumor 1 immunoreactivity excludes the possibility of serous carcinoma. (**A–G**), Hematoxylin and eosin staining; (**H–K**), immunohistochemical staining with polymer method. Original magnification: (**A**), 4×; (**B**), 40×; (**C**), 100×; (**D**), 20×; (**E**), 100×; (**F**), 200×; (**G**), 40×; (**H**), 60×; (**I**), 60×; (**J**), 60×; (**K**), 80×.

Case 2: The hysterectomy specimen incidentally showed an ECP (Figure 3A). A 19 mm elongated polyp arising in the endocervix had a 3-mm exophytic tumor protruding from the surface (Figure 3B). The tumor invaded the polyp stroma superficially, at a depth of 0.3 mm. Histologically, the EC involving ECP consisted predominantly of solid cellular sheets showing severe nuclear pleomorphism (grade 3 EC; Figure 3C), intermingled with mature squamous morules (squamous differentiation; Figure 3D). In contrast, the endometrial tumor was EC of grade 1 with mucinous differentiation (Figure 3E,F), measuring 20 mm at its largest dimension and 14 mm at its deepest invasion depth. Additionally, the patient had an ovarian mass, which was histologically compatible with grade 3 EC (Figure 3G). The presence of predominantly solid architecture (Figure 3H) and scattered areas of squamous differentiation (Figure 3I) was similar to the EC involving ECP. Moreover, the high-grade ovarian tumor, which extensively involved the pelvic and extrapelvic peritoneum, exhibited high-grade nuclear atypia, geographic necrosis, and substantial LVI. Immunohistochemical staining revealed that the EC involving ECP was negative for ER (Figure 3J) and PR (Figure 3K) but diffusely and strongly positive for p16 (Figure 3L). The immunophenotypes of the ovarian EC were identical to those of the EC involving ECP: a complete absence of ER (Figure 3M) and PR (Figure 3N) expression and uniform p16 positivity with strong staining intensity (Figure 3O). WT1 negativity in the ovarian tumor excluded high-grade serous carcinoma (Figure 3P). In contrast, endometrial EC demonstrated diffuse and strong nuclear expression for ER (Figure 3Q) and PR (Figure 3R). Patchy p16 positivity in the endometrial EC (Figure 3S) was different from intense and uniform p16 expression in the ovary and ECP. Based on the similar morphology and immunohistochemical staining results, the EC involving ECP was considered a metastatic lesion of the ovarian EC.

Case 3: Endocervical curettage revealed a few pieces of endocervical tissue showing cystically dilated glands, fibrous stroma, and endocervical tissue fragments (Figure 4A). An 11 mm ECP was involved with the superficially invading tumor at the polyp surface (Figure 4B). This tumor measured 4 mm at its greatest dimension and 0.3 mm at its deepest invasion depth (Figure 4C). Foci of endocervical glandular extension were occasionally noted (Figure 4D). A well-differentiated glandular proliferation was associated with stromal inflammatory reaction (Figure 4E), and the tumor cells exhibited nuclear hyperchromasia and mild pleomorphism (Figure 4F). Immunohistochemically, patchy p16 positivity eliminated the possibility of HPV-associated EAC (Figure 4G). Uniform estrogen receptor immunoreactivity with intense staining intensity supported the diagnosis of grade 1 EC (Figure 4H). The endometrial tumor was an 8 mm EC without myometrial invasion (Figure 4I). The degree of cytological and architectural atypia matched that of the EC involving ECP (Figure 4J). No remarkable lesion was identified in the cervix (Figure 3K).

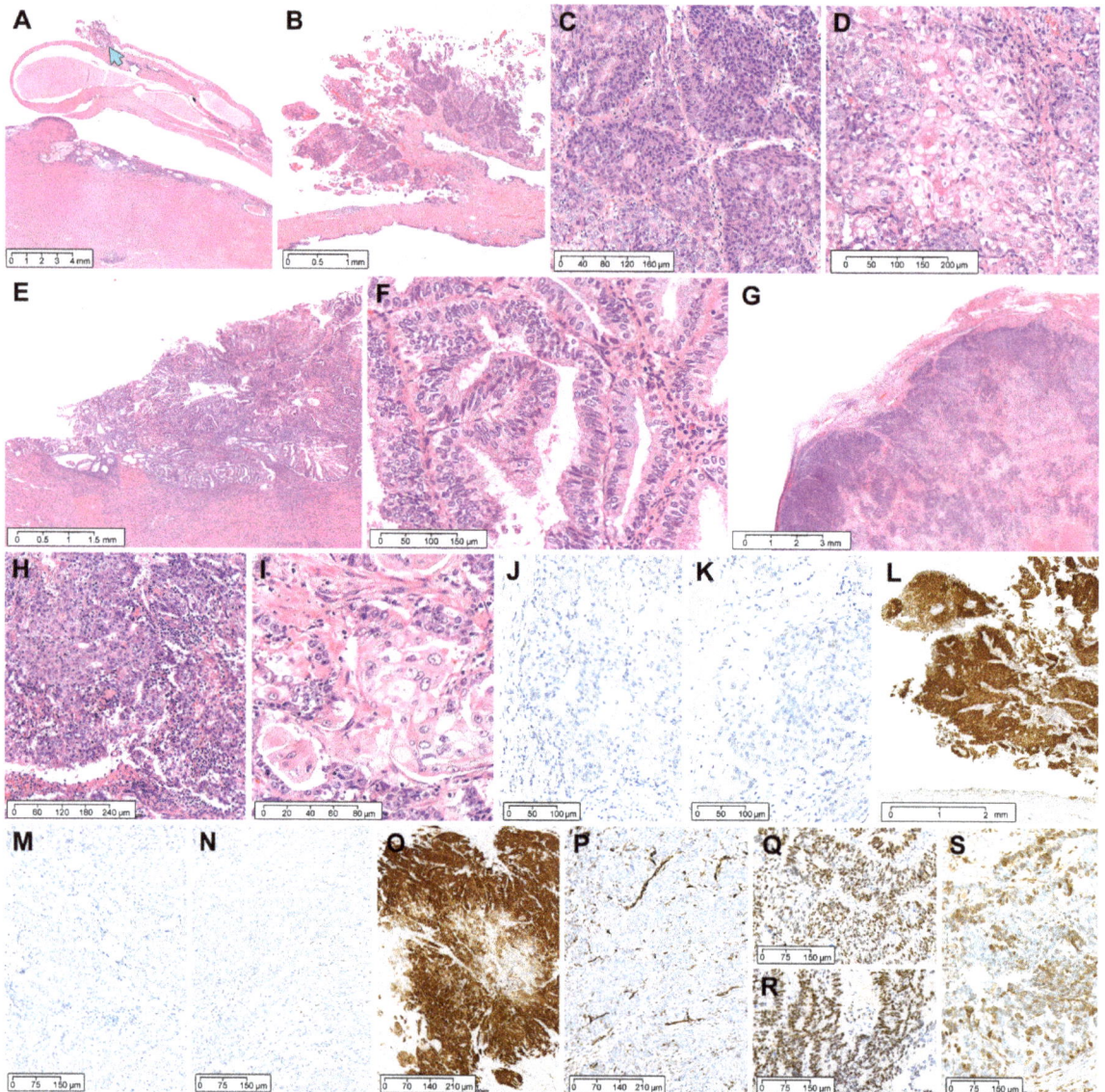

Figure 3. Grade 3 ovarian EC involving ECP: case 2. (**A**) The hysterectomy specimen shows an elongated ECP. EC (blue arrow) appears as an exophytic mass protruding from the surface of ECP. (**B**–**D**) EC involving ECP (**B**) superficially invades the stroma of the polyp up to 0.3 mm, (**C**) consists predominantly of solid sheets of tumor cells, and (**D**) exhibits severe nuclear pleomorphism, coarse chromatin, and prominent nucleoli. Foci of squamous differentiation are readily identifiable. (**E**) In the endometrial EC, well-differentiated glands are confluent and crowded. (**F**) Areas of mucinous differentiation are noted. (**G**) The ovarian EC demonstrates a diffuse infiltrative growth pattern with foci of geographic tumor necrosis. (**H**) The solid architecture occupies more than half of the tumor, compatible with grade 3 EC. (**I**) High-grade nuclear atypia and the presence of squamous differentiation are the same as those of EC involving ECP. (**J**–**S**) Immunohistochemically, EC involving ECP is negative for (**J**) estrogen receptor (ER) and (**K**) progesterone receptor (PR) and (**L**) positive for p16 with strong staining intensity. Ovarian EC is also negative for (**M**) ER and (**N**) PR and (**O**)

uniformly and intensely positive for p16. (**P**) WT1 negativity excludes the possibility of serous carcinoma. (**Q**–**S**) Endometrial EC shows strongly positive expression for (**Q**) ER and (**R**) PR and (**S**) patchy p16 positivity. (**A**–**I**), Hematoxylin and eosin staining. (**J**–**S**), immunohistochemical staining using polymer method. Original magnification: (**A**), 10×; (**B**), 20×; (**C**), 150×; (**D**), 200×; (**E**), 25×; (**F**), 200×; (**G**), 25×; (**H**), 100×; (**I**), 400×; (**J**), 150×; (**K**), 150×; (**L**), 30×; (**M**), 100×; (**N**), 100×; (**O**), 100×; (**P**), 100×; (**Q**), 100×; (**R**), 100×; (**S**), 100×.

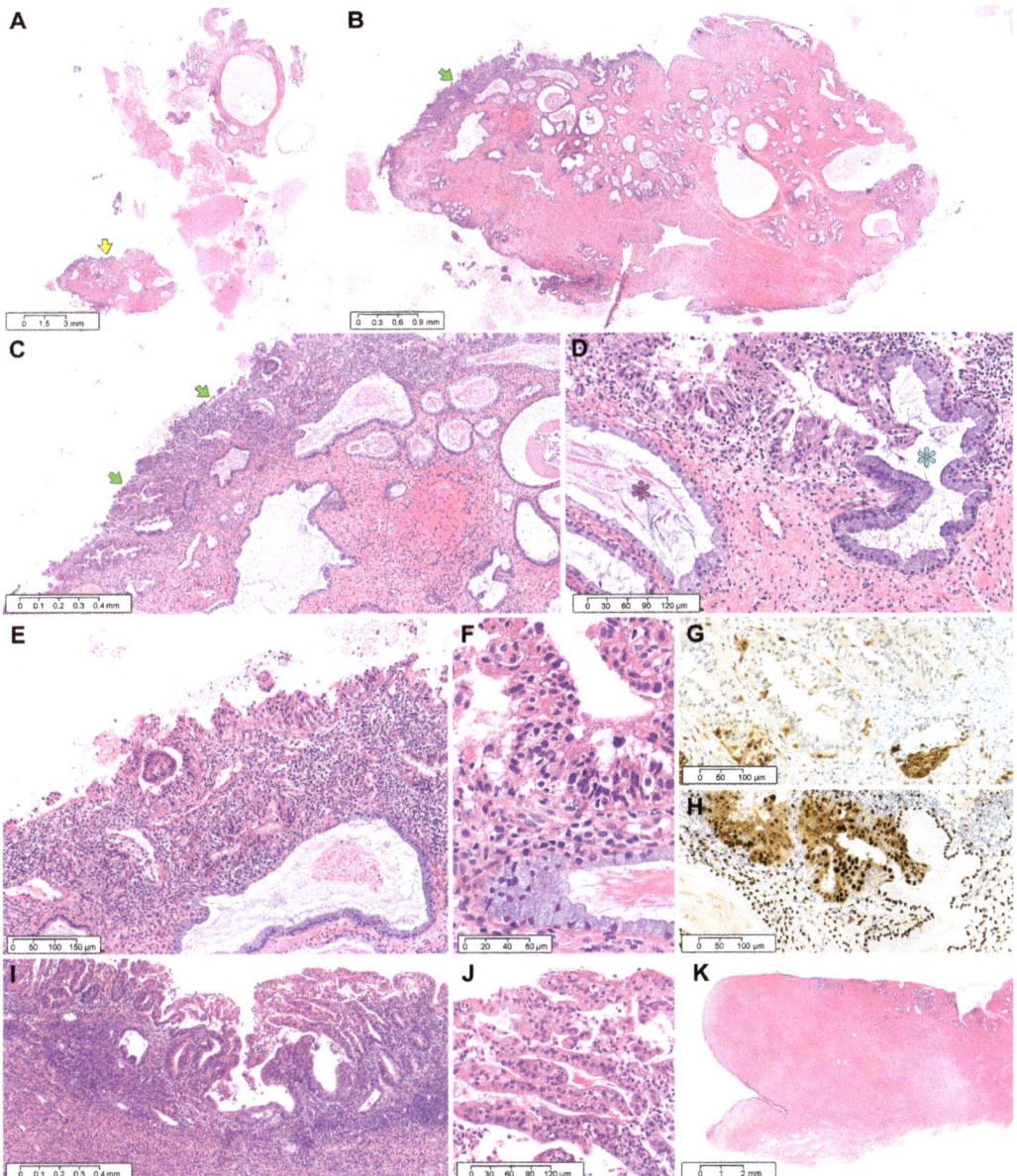

Figure 4. Grade 1 endometrial EC involving ECP: case 3. (**A**) The endocervical curettage specimen consists of fragmented ECP tissues, fibrin, and small endocervical tissues. One of the ECP fragments (yellow arrow) shows the tumor tissue. (**B**) The greatest dimension of EC involving the surface of

ECP measures 4 mm (green arrow). The presence of thick-walled blood vessels, fibrotic stroma, and an increased number of benign endocervical glands is characteristic of ECP. (**C**) The depth of invasion into the polyp stroma (green arrows) measures 0.3 mm. (**D**) The EC cells partially involve one endocervical gland (blue asterisk), in contrast to the other uninvolved one (purple asterisk). (**E**) The tumor is associated with a stromal inflammatory reaction. (**F**) On high-power magnification, compared with non-atypical endocervical gland (lower half), the EC cells (upper half) reveal nuclear enlargement, hyperchromasia, and loss of nuclear polarity. (**G**) Patchy p16 positivity rules out the possibility of human papillomavirus-associated endocervical adenocarcinoma. (**H**) Uniform nuclear estrogen receptor immunoreactivity with intense staining intensity supports the diagnosis of grade 1 EC. (**I**) Primary endometrial EC does not invade the myometrium. (**J**) The degree of nuclear atypia is the same as that of EC involving ECP. (**K**) The cervix shows no pathological abnormality. (**A–F**) and (**I–K**), Hematoxylin and eosin staining. (**G–H**), immunohistochemical staining using polymer method. Original magnification: (**A**), 2.5×; (**B**), 10×; (**C**), 40×; (**D**), 150×; (**E**), 100×; (**F**), 400×; (**G**), 100×; (**H**), 100×; (**I**), 40×; (**J**), 150×; (**K**), 4×.

Case 4: The polypectomy specimen revealed a 16 mm ovoid polyp with a short, slender stalk comprising a centrally dilated glandular lumen, peripherally stretched glands, and fibrotic stroma (Figure 5A). Complex and crowded glands were spread along the polyp surface (Figure 5B), and the superficial stroma of ECP was invaded by the tumor at a depth of 1 mm and a dimension of 10 mm. Endocervical glandular extension (Figure 5C) and stromal inflammatory infiltrates (Figure 5D) were present. The tumor cells displayed mild-to-moderate nuclear pleomorphism and enlargement (Figure 5E). Immunohistochemical staining revealed patchy p16 positivity (Figure 5F) and diffuse and strong expression for ER (Figure 5G) and PR (Figure 5H). The histological features were compatible with a grade 1 EC diagnosis. We found a 5-mm endometrial tumor without myometrial invasion or LVI. This endometrial lesion was morphologically (Figure 5I) and immunophenotypically (Figure 5J,K) identical to the EC involving ECP.

Table 3 summarizes the immunohistochemical staining results. The histological type of malignancy involving ECP was EC in all four cases, with two grade 3 ovarian ECs and three grade 1 endometrial ECs. One of the ovarian tumors exhibited foci of squamous differentiation, and one patient (case 2) had concomitant ovarian and endometrial ECs. Three cases displayed extension into the endocervical glands embedded in the polyp stroma. Although all tumors invaded the polyp stroma up to 1 mm of depth, no LVI was noted. The resection margin status was evaluated in two patients who underwent polypectomies. Both patients showed a negative resection margin, but the safety distance was < 1 mm in one case. No evidence of endometriosis, hyperplasia without atypia, or AH/EIN was observed in ECP, whereas all primary endometrial ECs were associated with AH/EIN and all ovarian tumors co-existed with endometriotic cysts. Interestingly, the three primary tumors (cases 1, 3, and 4) showed no LVI or lymph node metastasis. Detailed histopathological features of EC involving ECP are as follows.

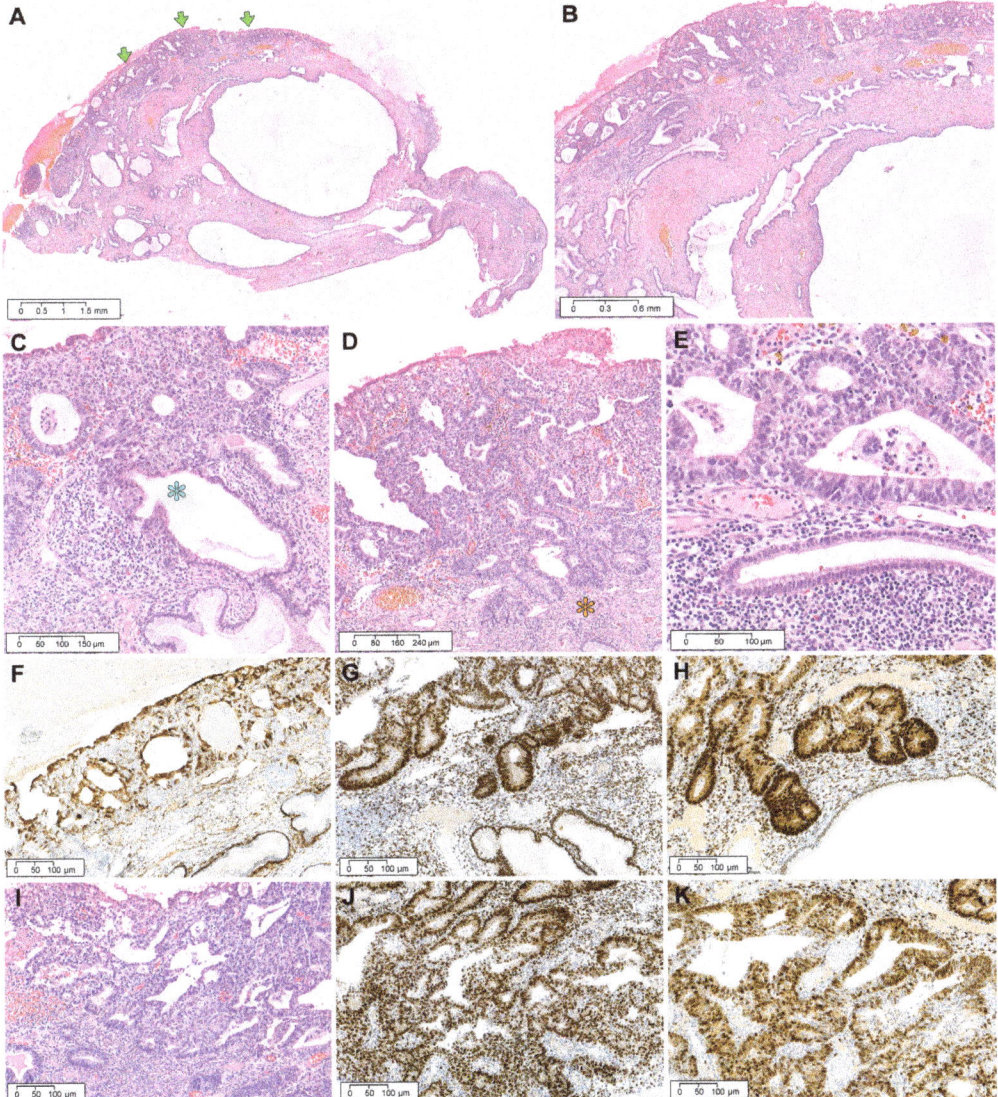

Figure 5. Grade 1 endometrial EC involving ECP: case 4. (**A**) The polypectomy specimen demonstrates the tumor tissue (green arrows) involving the surface. (**B**) Complex and crowded glandular architecture spreads along the surface and superficial stroma of ECP. (**C**) The EC cells partially involve one endocervical gland (blue asterisk). (**D**) Back-to-back arrangement (orange asterisk) and a lack of the intervening stroma are compatible with grade 1 EC. (**E**) High-power magnification reveals that the tumor glands (upper half) display nuclear stratification, enlargement, hyperchromasia, and loss of nuclear polarity. There is also a non-atypical endocervical gland (lower half). (**F–H**) Immunohistochemical staining reveals (**F**) patchy p16 positivity and diffuse and strong expression for (**G**) estrogen and (**H**) progesterone receptors. (**I–K**) Primary endometrial EC exhibits identical (**I**) histological features and immunoreactivities for (**J**) estrogen and (**K**) progesterone receptors to EC involving ECP. (**A–E**) and (**I**), Hematoxylin and eosin staining; (**F–H**), (**J**), and (**K**), immunohistochemical staining using polymer method. Original magnification: (**A**), 15×; (**B**), 20×; (**C**), 60×; (**D**), 40×; (**E**), 200×; (**F**), 100×; (**G**), 100×; (**H**), 100×; (**I**), 100×; (**J**), 100×; (**K**), 100×.

Table 3. The histological types and prevalence of gynecological tumors coexisting with ECP.

Case No	1		2			3		4	
	ECP	Ovary	ECP	Ovary	EM	ECP	EM	ECP	EM
ER	FSP	FSP	Neg	Neg	DSP	DSP	DSP	DSP	DSP
PR	FSP	FSP	Neg	Neg	DSP	FSP	FSP	DSP	DSP
p16	PP	PP	DSP	DSP	PP	PP	PP	PP	PP
p53	Mutant (CA)	Mutant (CA)	WT	WT	WT	WT	WT	WT	WT
Wilms tumor 1	Neg	Neg	Neg	Neg	Neg	NA	NA	NA	NA

CA: Complete absence; DSP: diffuse strong positive; ER: estrogen receptor; FSP: focal strong positive; Neg: negative; PP: patchy positive; PR: progesterone receptor; WT: wild type.

4. Discussion

To the best of our knowledge, no previous cases of the synchronous occurrence of endometrial or ovarian EC involving ECP have been reported. Our study described four such cases. In cases 3 and 4, we diagnosed EC involving ECP as a metastatic lesion from endometrial EC based on the following morphological features: (1) same histological features and immunohistochemical staining results between the EC involving ECP and the endometrium; (2) no involvement of the lower uterine segment and cervical stroma; (3) no LVI; (4) no precursor lesion (benign endometriosis and/or endometrial hyperplasia without atypia) in ECP; and (5) no premalignant lesion in ECP. Most endometrial ECs with the direct involvement of the cervix present as large tumors or with an epicenter in the lower uterine segment [31]. In some cases, the tumor cells spread to the endocervix along the surface or glandular epithelium. LVI is also one of the ways by which EC may involve the cervix. However, our two endometrial EC patients had no evidence of tumor involvement or LVI in the lower uterine segment, cervical stroma, and endocervical mucosa. EC of the uterine cervix is classified as one of the HPV-independent EACs according to the updated 2020 World Health Organization Classification [16]. Primary cervical EC may arise from benign endometriosis involving ECP and progress to AH/EIN and eventually EC. The absence of benign endometriosis, endometrial hyperplasia without atypia, or AH/EIN in ECP and adjacent non-polypoid endocervical tissue did not support the possibility of HPV-independent endometrioid-type EAC. Finally, we considered implantation metastasis as a possible mechanism of the ECP involvement of endometrial EC. Iatrogenic tumor implantation is a condition that results from various medical procedures used during the diagnosis or treatment of a malignancy [32]. In one study, of the 176 patients who underwent endometrial curettage before hysterectomy, 9 (5.1%) were found to have cervical implantation metastasis [33]. Moreover, endometrial carcinomas are well known to have an implantation capacity, which is the ability of tumor cells detached from the primary endometrial tumor to migrate to the peritoneal cavity through the fallopian tubes for implantation on the peritoneal surface, resulting in peritoneal, cervical, or vaginal implantation [34]. In a study by Stewart et al. [32], tumor cell emboli within the tubal lumina were identified in 26% and 3% of high- and low-grade endometrial carcinomas, respectively. Since we did not observe EC cells migrating through the endometrial cavity and endocervical canal experimentally, we could not clearly clarify the pathogenetic mechanism by which the endometrial EC involves ECP in this study. However, based on the absence of tumor involvement or LVI in the lower uterine segment, cervical stroma, and endocervical mucosa, the possibility that the tumor cells may have been implanted on the ECP surface through intrauterine migration can be considered. Even though our two endometrial EC patients had not undergone any previous diagnostic or therapeutic procedures prior to endocervical polypectomy (case 3) or endometrial curettage (case 4), it is reasonable to assume that the tumor cells may have adhered to the erosive and inflamed surface of the continuously compressed and irritated ECP within the narrow endocervical canal.

In cases 1 and 2, the histological features of the grade 3 EC involving ECP and the ovarian tumors were the same. Endometrial or cervical metastases of ovarian cancer are rarer than ovarian metastases of endometrial or cervical cancer [31,35]. Our finding of ovarian EC metastasizing to the ECP and spreading along the polyp surface or superficially invading into the polyp stroma appears to be novel. Substantial LVI was observed in case 2, whereas there was no LVI in the ovary and ECP in case 1. The latter case presented an unusual phenomenon, as the tumor cells must have migrated in the opposite direction, from the ovary and peritoneal cavity through the endometrium to the cervix. Ovarian EC cells on the ovarian surface or around fimbria may migrate through the tube and endometrial cavity to the endocervical canal [31,36]. Two cases of ovarian EC were initially advanced stage, with neoadjuvant chemotherapy being performed in one case. As a result of the pathological examination of the debulking specimen, both cases were stage IIIC and high-grade, and one (case 1) was p53-abnormal EC. In case 1, metastases to the sternum and rib occurred 49 months after post-operative adjuvant chemotherapy, and in case 2, metastasis was observed in the mesentery after three cycles of adjuvant chemotherapy. The presence of small metastases of ovarian EC to ECP less than 1 cm did not affect the treatment decisions or outcomes of the patients with the aggressive, advanced-stage, high-grade ovarian EC. Our findings did, however, reflect the high oncogenic aggressiveness shown in the migratory and metastatic ability of these tumors.

Case 2 demonstrated concurrent endometrial and ovarian ECs and multiple metastatic lesions in the abdominopelvic peritoneum and small bowel. The following differential diagnoses were initially considered: (1) adnexal and peritoneal involvement of endometrial cancer, (2) peritoneal and endometrial involvement of ovarian cancer, and (3) synchronous endometrial and ovarian cancers with peritoneal extension from either endometrium or ovary. The histology (high-grade EC with squamous differentiation) and immunophenotype (hormone receptor negativity and diffuse, strong p16 positivity) of the peritoneal metastatic lesions were the same as those of the ovarian tumors. However, the endometrial tumors were low-grade EC with mucinous differentiation, showing uniform hormone receptor positivity and p16 patchy positivity. Based on these results, it was determined that the possibility of synchronous stage IIIC ovarian cancer (with extrapelvic peritoneal metastases) and stage IB endometrial cancers was high. The EC observed in ECP also had the same morphology and immunophenotype as the ovarian EC but were different from the endometrial EC. Additionally, endometriosis, endometrial hyperplasia without atypia, and AH/EIN, suggesting the possibility of primary HPV-independent endometrioid-type EAC, were absent in ECP. Therefore, the EC involving ECP was reasonably considered a metastasis of the ovarian EC.

Several clinical implications of the involvement of ECP by endometrial or ovarian EC were considered. First, in case 3, grade 1 EC involving ECP was diagnosed in the curettage of an incidentally detected endocervical mass. In case 4, grade 1 EC was found in an endocervical polypectomy specimen, although an endometrial lesion was not suspected clinically. As in these cases, when metastatic tumors involving ECP were first detected where the primary endometrial EC was not known, the lesions helped detect endometrial cancer at the early stages. Second, in cases 3 and 4, where EC invaded the polyp stroma to a depth of less than 1 mm, the lesions could not be considered cervical stromal extensions, a FIGO stage II finding of endometrial cancer. In other words, adjuvant radiation therapy, the standard treatment for stage II endometrial cancer, was not required. The treatment could differ, in the case of case 3 potentially being misinterpreted as an endometrioid-type EAC involving ECP, for instance. The gynecologists may have considered whether to perform radical hysterectomy with bilateral salpingo-oophorectomy and pelvic lymph node dissection, the standard treatment for cervical cancer, or simply a total hysterectomy with bilateral salpingo-oophorectomy, considering that there was no visible uterine lesion and lymph node metastasis on MRI. Third, when stratified according to the stage, grade, and myometrial invasion, no statistically significant differences in the recurrence rate between patients with or without cervical implantation metastasis exist [33], indicating that cervical implantation metastasis does not appear to alter prognoses or require specific treatment. In this study, since the ovarian ECs of cases 1 and 2 were advanced-stage diseases, the ECP tumor did not affect the treatment. In addition, the ECP involvement by endometrial EC in cases 3 and 4 did not affect the treatment guideline in these cases, as the ECP was removed with the total hysterectomies.

Differential diagnoses of EC involving ECP include reactive endocervical lesions, including squamous metaplasia (SM) and microglandular hyperplasia (MGH), and HPV-associated usual-type EAC. ECPs are commonly accompanied by SM, MGH, and chronic inflammation. Immature SM is characterized by evenly spaced, small, round nuclei and dense, scant cytoplasm involving the superficial epithelium and glands of ECP. Case 1 revealed SM involving ECP on the non-neoplastic areas of the polyp (Figure 6A–C). SM had no mitotic activity or significant nuclear or architectural atypia (Figure 6D). The intervening stroma displayed fibrosis and chronic inflammation (Figure 6E). MGH consists of closely packed, small glands with mucin-containing epithelium in the background of mildly inflamed stroma. Despite a compact glandular proliferation, MGH exhibits no nuclear pleomorphism or architectural abnormality. HPV-associated usual-type EAC is the most common type of EAC, with apical mitoses and apoptotic bodies readily identifiable by scanning or low-power magnification. Block p16 positivity is the hallmark of HPV-associated EAC, but all our cases showed patchy p16 immunoreactivity.

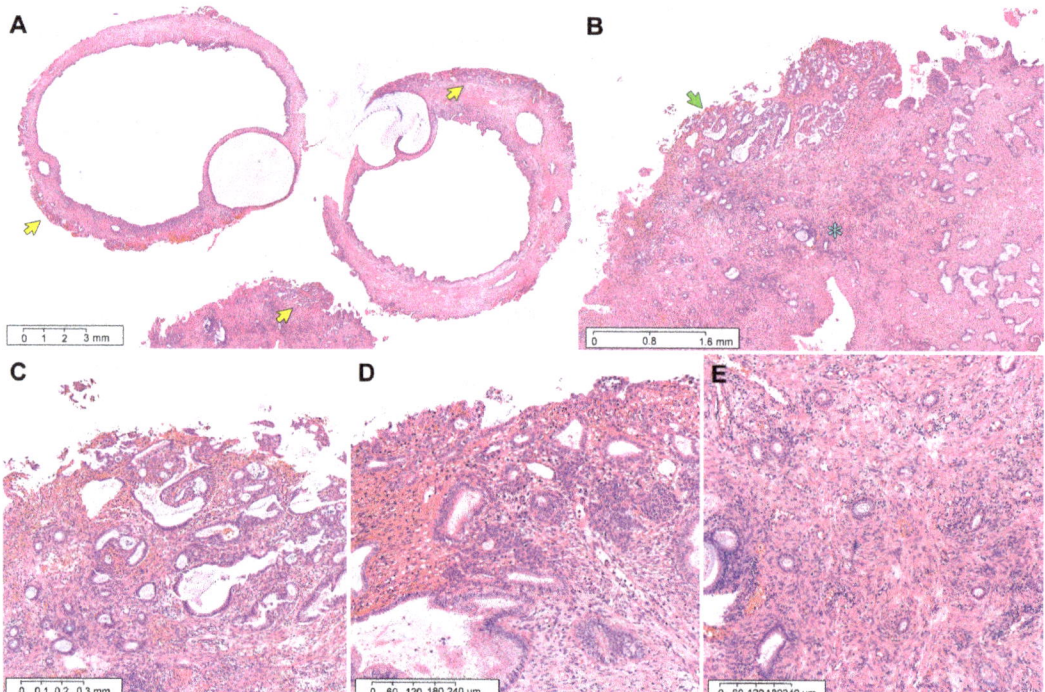

Figure 6. SM involving ECP. (**A**) ECP of case 1 reveals areas of SM and reactive glandular proliferation (yellow arrows). Some cystically dilated glands are present. (**B**) In addition to the immature SM (green arrow), small glands are embedded in the fibrotic stroma (blue asterisk). (**C**) The endocervical glands in SM lesions vary in size and shape. (**D**) Metaplastic squamous epithelium possesses small, bland nuclei and scant cytoplasm and grows beneath the pre-existing endocervical epithelium. There is no complex glandular proliferation, solid architecture, cribriforming, or high-grade cytological atypia. (**E**) The stroma exhibits fibrosis and mixed chronic inflammatory infiltrates. (**A**–**E**), Hematoxylin and eosin staining. Original magnification: (**A**), 15×; (**B**), 40×; (**C**), 100×; (**D**), 150×; (**E**), 120×.

5. Conclusions

In summary, we evaluated the histological types and prevalence of gynecological tumors co-existing with ECP. We observed that 69 of the 429 ECPs (15.9%) were found to be associated with premalignant or malignant lesions of the uterine cervix, endometrium, and ovary. Of these, four (0.9%) ECPs were involved by endometrial or ovarian ECs. We investigated the clinicopathological characteristics of the four cases of ECP that were involved by EC. In two cases of ovarian EC, EC involving ECP exhibited similar morphology and immunohistochemical staining results as those of advanced-stage ovarian EC. In two cases of endometrial EC, the histological and immunophenotypical features of the EC involving ECP were identical to those of the primary endometrial tumor, despite the lack of tumor involvement in the myometrium, lower uterine segment, and cervical stroma as well as the absence of LVI and lymph node metastasis. In all cases, no evidence of benign endometriosis, endometrial hyperplasia without atypia, or AH/EIN within ECP or the adjacent endocervical tissue was noted. Based on clinical history, histological features, and immunohistochemical staining results, we concluded that they were metastatic from the endometrial or ovarian ECs, as possible implantation metastases. The determination of the type and origin of metastatic tumors is an important and potentially challenging area in pathology, as it affects the clinical decision and patient management. The site of origin is best determined by correlating clinical and pathologic findings. The occurrence of endometrial and ovarian carcinomas metastatic to ECPs is a rare phenomenon. To the best of our knowledge, we described the first synchronous occurrence of EC involving ECP and endometrial or ovarian EC. Awareness of these unusual phenomena is vital in proper diagnosis and clinical practices.

Author Contributions: Conceptualization, J.S., Y.L. and H.-S.K.; methodology, J.S.; validation, Y.L.; investigation, J.S.; resources, H.-S.K.; data curation, Y.L.; writing—original draft preparation, J.S. and H.-S.K.; writing—review and editing, Y.L. and H.-S.K.; visualization, H.-S.K.; supervision, H.-S.K. All authors have read and agreed to the published version of the manuscript.

Funding: This research received no external funding.

Institutional Review Board Statement: The study was approved by the Institutional Review Board of Samsung Medical Center (protocol code: 2022-07-048; date of approval: 11 July 2022).

Informed Consent Statement: Written informed consent has been obtained from the patients to publish this paper.

Data Availability Statement: Not applicable.

Conflicts of Interest: The authors declare no conflict of interest.

References

1. Park, C.K.; Kim, Y.W.; Koh, H.H.; Yoon, N.; Bae, G.E.; Kim, H.S. Clinicopathological characteristics of squamous cell carcinoma and high-grade squamous intraepithelial lesions involving endocervical polyps. *In Vivo* **2020**, *34*, 2613–2621. [CrossRef] [PubMed]
2. Misugi, T.; Kitada, K.; Fudaba, M.; Tanaka, S.; Kurihara, Y.; Tahara, M.; Hamuro, A.; Nakano, A.; Koyama, M.; Tachibana, D. Preliminary outcomes of cervical cerclage for shortened cervix with decidual polyp. *Healthcare* **2022**, *10*, 1312. [CrossRef] [PubMed]
3. Park, S.; Bae, G.E.; Kim, J.; Kim, H.S. Mesonephric-like differentiation of endometrial endometrioid carcinoma: Clinicopathological and molecular characteristics distinct from those of uterine mesonephric-like adenocarcinoma. *Diagnostics* **2021**, *11*, 1450. [CrossRef] [PubMed]
4. Alexandrova, E.; Pecoraro, G.; Sellitto, A.; Melone, V.; Ferravante, C.; Rocco, T.; Guacci, A.; Giurato, G.; Nassa, G.; Rizzo, F.; et al. An overview of candidate therapeutic target genes in ovarian cancer. *Cancers* **2020**, *12*, 1470. [CrossRef]
5. Anglesio, M.S.; Yong, P.J. Endometriosis-associated ovarian cancers. *Clin. Obs. Gynecol.* **2017**, *60*, 711–727. [CrossRef]
6. Noe, M.; Ayhan, A.; Wang, T.L.; Shih, I.M. Independent development of endometrial epithelium and stroma within the same endometriosis. *J. Pathol.* **2018**, *245*, 265–269. [CrossRef]
7. Assem, H.; Rambau, P.F.; Lee, S.; Ogilvie, T.; Sienko, A.; Kelemen, L.E.; Kobel, M. High-grade endometrioid carcinoma of the ovary: A clinicopathologic study of 30 cases. *Am. J. Surg. Pathol.* **2018**, *42*, 534–544. [CrossRef]

8. Bennett, J.A.; Pesci, A.; Morales-Oyarvide, V.; Da Silva, A.; Nardi, V.; Oliva, E. Incidence of mismatch repair protein deficiency and associated clinicopathologic features in a cohort of 104 ovarian endometrioid carcinomas. *Am. J. Surg. Pathol.* **2019**, *43*, 235–243. [CrossRef]
9. Choi, K.H.; Kim, H.; Bae, G.E.; Lee, S.H.; Woo, H.Y.; Kim, H.S. Mesonephric-like differentiation of ovarian endometrioid and high-grade serous carcinomas: Clinicopathological and molecular characteristics distinct from those of mesonephric-like adenocarcinoma. *Anticancer Res.* **2021**, *41*, 4587–4601. [CrossRef]
10. Seay, K.; Bustamante, B.; Khutti, S.; Frimer, M. A case of non-HPV related primary endometrioid adenocarcinoma of the cervix. *Gynecol. Oncol. Rep.* **2020**, *32*, 100579. [CrossRef]
11. Ren, H.; Almadani, N.; Pors, J.; Leung, S.; Ho, J.; Chow, C.; Ta, M.; Park, K.J.; Stolnicu, S.; Soslow, R.; et al. International Endocervical Adenocarcinoma Criteria and Classification (IECC): An independent cohort with clinical and molecular findings. *Int. J. Gynecol. Pathol.* **2021**, *40*, 533–540. [CrossRef]
12. Hodgson, A.; Park, K.J.; Djordjevic, B.; Howitt, B.E.; Nucci, M.R.; Oliva, E.; Stolnicu, S.; Xu, B.; Soslow, R.A.; Parra-Herran, C. International Endocervical Adenocarcinoma Criteria and Classification: Validation and interobserver reproducibility. *Am. J. Surg. Pathol.* **2019**, *43*, 75–83. [CrossRef]
13. Stolnicu, S.; Barsan, I.; Hoang, L.; Patel, P.; Terinte, C.; Pesci, A.; Aviel-Ronen, S.; Kiyokawa, T.; Alvarado-Cabrero, I.; Pike, M.C.; et al. International Endocervical Adenocarcinoma Criteria and Classification (IECC): A new pathogenetic classification for invasive adenocarcinomas of the endocervix. *Am. J. Surg. Pathol.* **2018**, *42*, 214–226. [CrossRef]
14. Gilks, C.B.; Kommoss, F. Synchronous tumours of the female reproductive tract. *Pathology* **2018**, *50*, 214–221. [CrossRef]
15. Amant, F.; Mirza, M.R.; Koskas, M.; Creutzberg, C.L. Cancer of the corpus uteri. *Int. J. Gynaecol. Obs.* **2018**, *143* (Suppl. S2), 37–50. [CrossRef]
16. WHO Classification of Tumors Editorial Board. *WHO Classification of Tumours: Female Genital Tumours*; IARC: Lyon, France, 2020.
17. Choi, S.; Na, K.; Kim, S.W.; Kim, H.S. Dedifferentiated mesonephric-like adenocarcinoma of the uterine corpus. *Anticancer Res.* **2021**, *41*, 2719–2726. [CrossRef]
18. Jung, H.; Bae, G.E.; Kim, H.M.; Kim, H.S. Clinicopathological and molecular differences between gastric-type mucinous carcinoma and usual-type endocervical adenocarcinoma of the uterine cervix. *Cancer Genom. Proteom.* **2020**, *17*, 627–641. [CrossRef]
19. Koh, H.H.; Jung, Y.Y.; Kim, H.S. Clinicopathological characteristics of gastric-type endocervical adenocarcinoma misdiagnosed as an endometrial, ovarian or extragenital malignancy, or mistyped as usual-type endocervical adenocarcinoma. *In Vivo* **2021**, *35*, 2261–2273. [CrossRef]
20. Lee, J.; Park, S.; Woo, H.Y.; Kim, H.S. Clinicopathological characteristics of microscopic tubal intraepithelial metastases from adenocarcinoma and small cell neuroendocrine carcinoma of the uterine cervix. *In Vivo* **2021**, *35*, 2469–2481. [CrossRef]
21. Park, S.; Kim, H.S. Primary retroperitoneal mucinous carcinoma with carcinosarcomatous mural nodules: A case report with emphasis on its histological features and immunophenotype. *Diagnostics* **2020**, *10*, 580. [CrossRef]
22. Yoon, N.; Kim, H.S.; Lee, J.W.; Lee, E.J.; Maeng, L.S.; Yoon, W.S. Targeted genomic sequencing reveals different evolutionary patterns between locally and distally recurrent glioblastomas. *Cancer Genom. Proteom.* **2020**, *17*, 803–812. [CrossRef]
23. Choi, S.; Cho, J.; Lee, S.E.; Baek, C.H.; Kim, Y.K.; Kim, H.J.; Ko, Y.H. Adenocarcinoma of the minor salivary gland with concurrent *MAML2* and *EWSR1* alterations. *J. Pathol. Transl. Med.* **2021**, *55*, 132–138. [CrossRef]
24. Choi, S.; Joo, J.W.; Do, S.I.; Kim, H.S. Endometrium-limited metastasis of extragenital malignancies: A challenge in the diagnosis of endometrial curettage specimens. *Diagnostics* **2020**, *10*, 150. [CrossRef]
25. Choi, S.; Jung, Y.Y.; Kim, H.S. Serous carcinoma of the endometrium with mesonephric-like differentiation initially misdiagnosed as uterine mesonephric-like adenocarcinoma: A case report with emphasis on the immunostaining and the identification of splice site *TP53* mutation. *Diagnostics* **2021**, *11*, 717. [CrossRef]
26. Choi, S.; Park, S.; Chung, M.P.; Kim, T.S.; Cho, J.H.; Han, J. A rare case of adenosquamous carcinoma arising in the background of IgG4-related lung disease. *J. Pathol. Transl. Med.* **2019**, *53*, 188–191. [CrossRef]
27. Jang, Y.; Jung, H.; Kim, H.N.; Seo, Y.; Alsharif, E.; Nam, S.J.; Kim, S.W.; Lee, J.E.; Park, Y.H.; Cho, E.Y.; et al. Clinicopathologic characteristics of HER2-positive pure mucinous carcinoma of the breast. *J. Pathol. Transl. Med.* **2020**, *54*, 95–102. [CrossRef]
28. Kim, H.; Kim, J.; Lee, S.K.; Cho, E.Y.; Cho, S.Y. TFE3-expressing perivascular epithelioid cell tumor of the breast. *J. Pathol. Transl. Med.* **2019**, *53*, 62–65. [CrossRef]
29. Kwon, H.J.; Song, S.Y.; Kim, H.S. Prominent papillary growth pattern and severe nuclear pleomorphism induced by neoadjuvant chemotherapy in ovarian mucinous carcinoma: Potential for misdiagnosis as high-grade serous carcinoma. *Anticancer Res.* **2021**, *41*, 1579–1586. [CrossRef]
30. Kobel, M.; Ronnett, B.M.; Singh, N.; Soslow, R.A.; Gilks, C.B.; McCluggage, W.G. Interpretation of p53 immunohistochemistry in endometrial carcinomas: Toward increased reproducibility. *Int. J. Gynecol. Pathol.* **2019**, *38*, S123–S131. [CrossRef]
31. McCluggage, W.G.; Hurrell, D.P.; Kennedy, K. Metastatic carcinomas in the cervix mimicking primary cervical adenocarcinoma and adenocarcinoma in situ: Report of a series of cases. *Am. J. Surg. Pathol.* **2010**, *34*, 735–741. [CrossRef]
32. Stewart, C.J.; Doherty, D.A.; Havlat, M.; Koay, M.H.; Leung, Y.C.; Naran, A.; O'Brien, D.; Ruba, S.; Salfinger, S.; Tan, J. Transtubal spread of endometrial carcinoma: Correlation of intra-luminal tumour cells with tumour grade, peritoneal fluid cytology, and extra-uterine metastasis. *Pathology* **2013**, *45*, 382–387. [CrossRef] [PubMed]
33. Fanning, J.; Alvarez, P.M.; Tsukada, Y.; Piver, M.S. Cervical implantation metastasis by endometrial adenocarcinoma. *Cancer* **1991**, *68*, 1335–1339. [CrossRef]

34. Wang, Y.; Du, J.; Lv, S.; Sui, Y.; Xue, X.; Sun, C.; Zou, J.; Ma, Q.; Fu, G.; Song, Q.; et al. Vaginal implantation metastasis of endometrial carcinoma: A case report. *Oncol. Lett.* **2016**, *12*, 513–515. [CrossRef] [PubMed]
35. Malpica, A.; Deavers, M.T. Ovarian low-grade serous carcinoma involving the cervix mimicking a cervical primary. *Int. J. Gynecol. Pathol.* **2011**, *30*, 613–619. [CrossRef]
36. Stewart, C.J.R.; Crum, C.P.; McCluggage, W.G.; Park, K.J.; Rutgers, J.K.; Oliva, E.; Malpica, A.; Parkash, V.; Matias-Guiu, X.; Ronnett, B.M. Guidelines to aid in the distinction of endometrial and endocervical carcinomas, and the distinction of independent primary carcinomas of the endometrium and adnexa from metastatic spread between these and other sites. *Int. J. Gynecol. Pathol.* **2019**, *38* (Suppl. S1), S75–S92. [CrossRef]

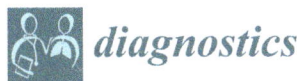

Interesting Images

Clear-Cell Mesothelioma of Uterine Corpus: Diagnostic Challenges in Intraoperative Frozen Sections

Tip Pongsuvareeyakul [1,*], Kanokkan Saipattranusorn [2], Kornkanok Sukpan [1], Prapaporn Suprasert [3] and Surapan Khunamornpong [1]

1. Department of Pathology, Faculty of Medicine, Chiang Mai University, Chiang Mai 50200, Thailand
2. Department of Pathology, Chonburi Hospital, Chonburi 20000, Thailand
3. Department of Obstetrics and Gynecology, Faculty of Medicine, Chiang Mai University, Chiang Mai 50200, Thailand
* Correspondence: tang_tip@hotmail.com

Abstract: The clear-cell variant of epithelioid mesothelioma is an extremely rare neoplasm of the peritoneum. It shares histomorphologic features overlapping with a wide variety of tumors including carcinomas and other non-epithelial neoplasms. The diagnosis of peritoneal clear-cell mesothelioma is not always straightforward, despite known immunohistochemistry (IHC) markers. Due to its rarity, this entity may be diagnostically confused with other clear-cell neoplasms, particularly in intraoperative frozen sections. Here, we present a case of clear-cell mesothelioma originating in the uterine serosa that was initially misdiagnosed as clear-cell adenocarcinoma in the intraoperative frozen section. Microscopically, the tumor showed diffuse tubulocystic spaces of variable size lined by clear cells with moderate nuclear atypia. Immunohistochemical staining confirmed the diagnosis of clear-cell mesothelioma. Recognition of this entity, albeit rare, is important as the diagnosis may significantly affect the management considerations. The judicious use of an IHC panel helps to distinguish this tumor from other mimickers.

Keywords: clear-cell mesothelioma; peritoneum; clear-cell carcinoma; frozen section; uterus

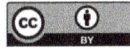

Table 1. Malignant mesothelioma of the peritoneum in women is 3.5 times less common than the pleural counterpart [1]. The incidence rate of peritoneal mesothelioma is only 0.1 per 100,000 women [2]. The differential diagnosis of peritoneal mesothelioma includes a wide variety of malignant tumors in contrast to pleural mesothelioma, which should be distinguished from pulmonary adenocarcinoma in the majority of cases [3]. Peritoneal mesothelioma has clinical, morphological, and molecular features that are distinctive from the pleural counterpart [4] (this table). It occurs more commonly in young women, and the association with asbestos exposure is much less strong than that of pleural mesothelioma [4]. In a large study of 164 cases of peritoneal mesothelioma in women [2], 40 cases (24.4%) had an initial referral diagnosis of Mullerian-type carcinomas or non-gynecological carcinomas. The large majority of tumors had epithelioid morphology (80.5%), whereas the remainder (19.5%) had biphasic morphology (epithelioid and sarcomatoid). Mixed architectural patterns were observed in 92% of cases, including papillary, solid, tubular or glandular, single-cell, and cystic patterns. The presence of clear cells or hobnail cells was found in a minority of cases (number not specified) [2]. Clear-cell mesothelioma represents an extremely rare subtype of peritoneal mesothelioma [5]. As the tumor shows clear cytoplasmic features, the histomorphology is overlapping with Mullerian clear-cell adenocarcinoma of the female genital organs. In this report, we describe a case of clear-cell mesothelioma originating in the uterine serosa. The morphological features of this tumor closely mimic clear-cell adenocarcinoma, resulting in an incorrect intraoperative frozen section diagnosis, which affected the surgical management decision. Comparison of clinico-pathological features of mesothelioma [1,2,4,6–15].

Table 1. Cont.

Clinico-Pathological Features	Pleural Mesothelioma	Peritoneal Mesothelioma	Peritoneal Clear-Cell Mesothelioma
Male: Female ratio	3.9:1	1.3:1	Female
Median age (years)	65–70	49–69 (49 in female) a	Limited data
Association with asbestos exposure	70%	33% (5–23% in female) a	Limited data
Association with germline cancer susceptibility mutations	7%	25%	Limited data
Histologic patterns	Epithelioid (55%) Biphasic (20%) Sarcomatoid (10%)	Epithelioid (82%) Biphasic (13%) Sarcomatoid (5%)	Epithelioid (limited data)
Loss of BAP1 immunoexpression b	80%a (especially epithelioid type)	57% a	Limited data
Median overall survival time (months)	17–20	53	Limited data

a Data in female patients. b Surrogate marker for BAP1 mutation.

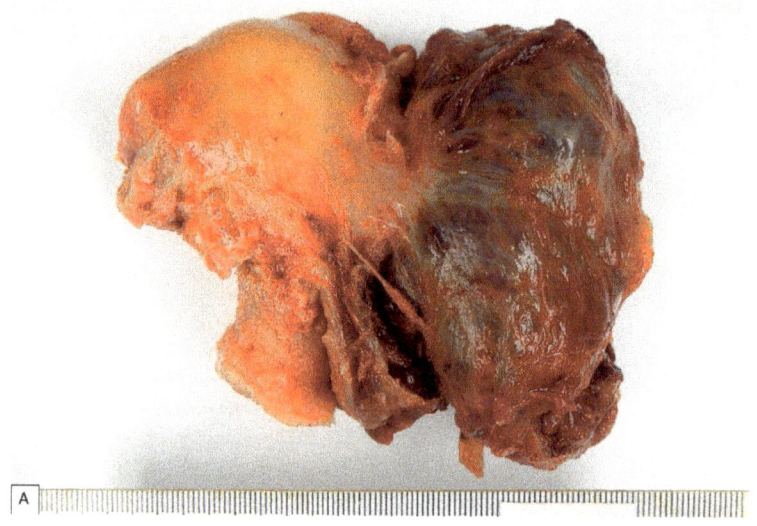

Figure 1. Cont.

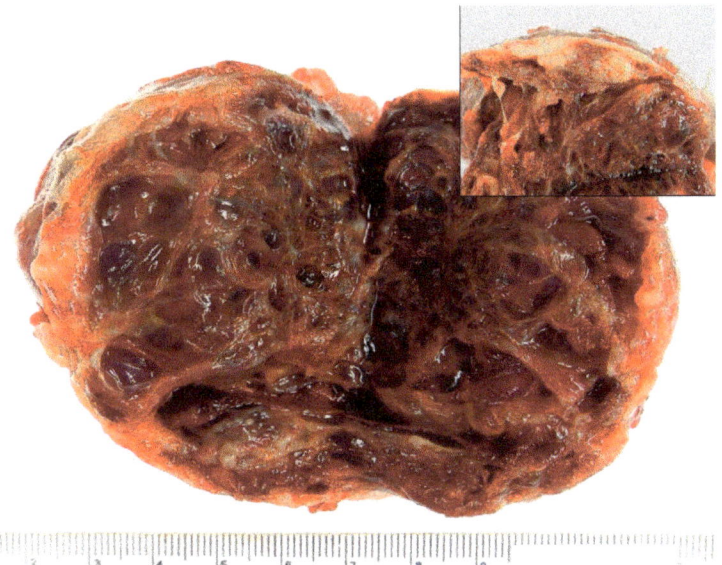

Figure 1. A 28-year-old Thai pregnant woman underwent an uneventful cesarean section at a local hospital. A 6 cm mass, right lateral to the uterus, was incidentally found. Follow-up computed tomography of the whole abdomen showed a 9.1 cm cystic mass with irregularly thick septation in the right adnexal region, consistent with an ovarian tumor. The patient was referred to Maharaj Nakorn Chiang Mai Hospital for further management two months after delivery. The patient had no clinical history of asbestos exposure or underlying diseases. Her family history was unremarkable. Preoperative laboratory investigations revealed a slight elevation of the CA125 tumor marker (70.6 U/mL; normal 0–35 U/mL). Intraoperatively, a large tumor protruding from uterine serosa was seen. Total abdominal hysterectomy was performed, and the uterus was sent for an intraoperative frozen section. Macroscopically, a 9 × 7 × 5.5 cm serosal tumor was found at the right posterolateral wall, as presented in (**A**). Cut surface of the tumor was dark red and revealed predominantly thin-walled multicystic to spongy tissue containing blood, as presented in (**B**), with focal tan solid area at the periphery ((**B**), **inset**). Frozen section diagnosis was clear-cell adenocarcinoma involving uterine serosa. Then, the patient underwent a complete surgical staging procedure, including bilateral salpingo-oophorectomy (BSO), bilateral pelvic node biopsy, omental biopsy, and peritoneal washing. Such intraoperative diagnosis was the main reason for complete surgical staging including immediate BSO and lymphadenectomy, which may not be the necessary surgical procedure for mesothelioma in young women in whom preservation of ovarian function is of concern. This figure and Figure 2 demonstrate the macroscopic and microscopic appearance of clear-cell mesothelioma that has led to the intraoperative diagnosis of clear-cell adenocarcinoma. The occurrence of extragenital clear-cell adenocarcinoma, although uncommon, could be expected, as clear-cell adenocarcinoma is common in the Eastern world, accounting for up to 27% of ovarian epithelial cancers in Japan [6], and this tumor can arise from non-ovarian endometriosis. While the diagnosis of clear-cell adenocarcinoma in the endometrium or the ovary may not require or depend on immunohistochemistry, the diagnosis of clear-cell adenocarcinoma of peritoneal origin needs to be supported by an appropriate and extensive immunohistochemical panel. The differential diagnoses of clear-cell mesothelioma include Mullerian-type adenocarcinomas with clear-cell features, non-Mullerian clear-cell carcinomas with relatively occult origin (e.g., clear-cell renal cell carcinoma), and other non-epithelial clear-cell neoplasms.

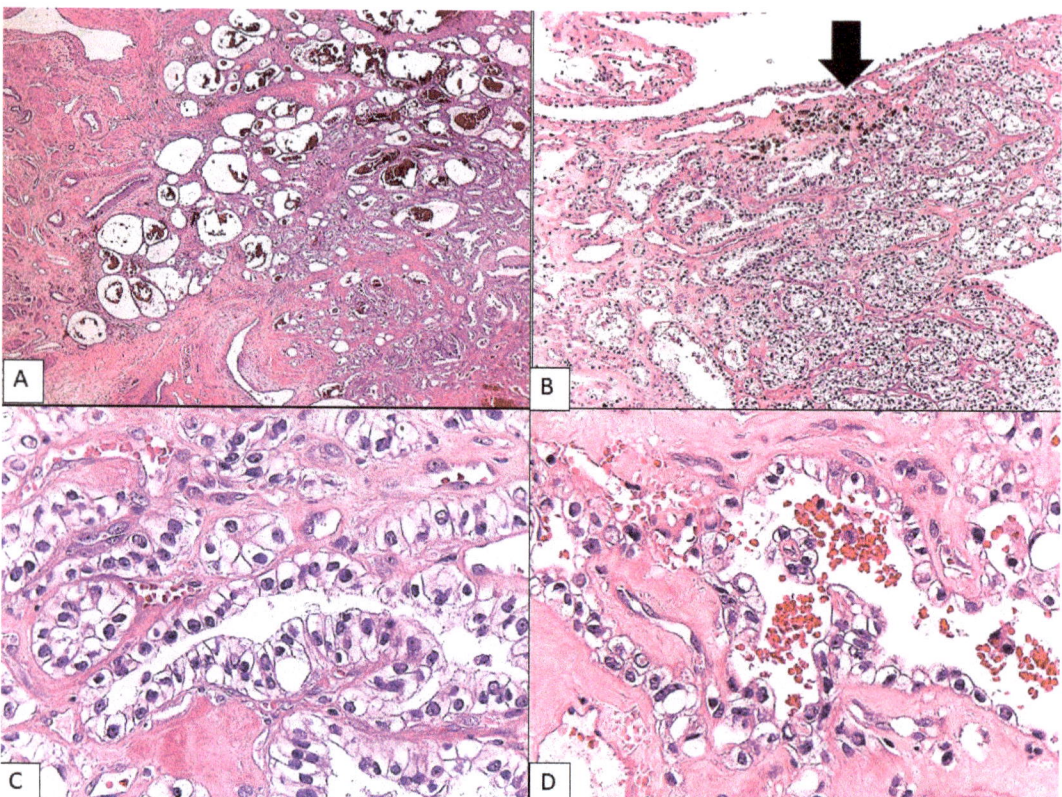

Figure 2. Histologic findings of clear-cell mesothelioma. The tumor showed an infiltrative border involving the outer myometrial wall (**A**) (**H&E, 40×**). The tumor was composed of diffuse tubulocystic spaces of varying size lined by monotonously uniform clear cells (**B**) (**H&E, 100×**). These cells exhibited abundant clear cytoplasm and hyperchromatic nuclei with moderate atypia and occasional distinct nucleoli (**C**) (**H&E, 400×**) or had a hobnail appearance (**D**) (**H&E, 400×**). Mitoses were rare (<1 in 10 high power fields). Scattered hemorrhage and hemosiderin deposits were present in fibrous septa ((**B**), **arrow**), but endometriosis was not identified. The tubulocystic pattern of this tumor is indistinguishable from that of clear-cell adenocarcinoma. However, the tumor lacks other common features of clear-cell adenocarcinoma including papillary architecture, hyalinized stromal material, adenofibromatous component, and the association with endometriotic focus. The absence of these features and the extraovarian location led to serious consideration for other tumors with clear-cell morphology. In the absence of a clinically identifiable primary site in any visceral organs, the exclusion of mesothelioma is necessary.

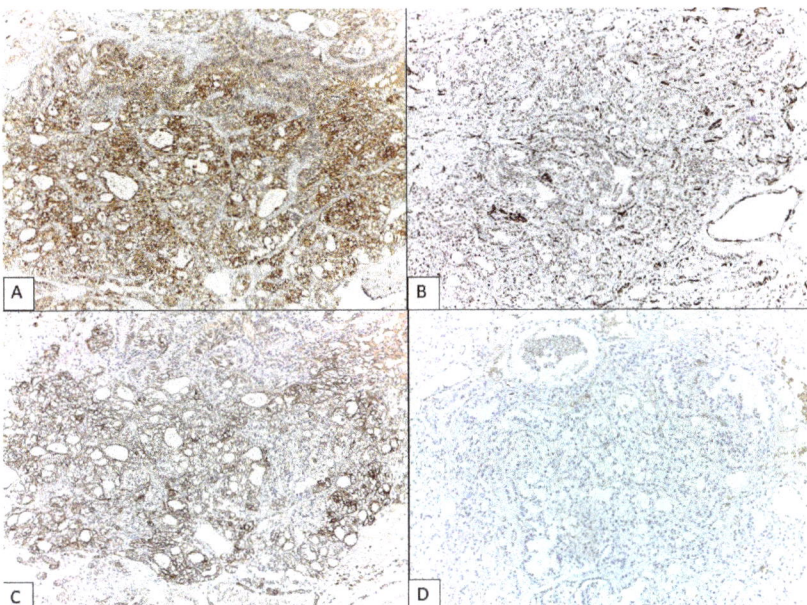

Figure 3. Immunohistochemical profile of clear-cell mesothelioma. Diffuse immunopositivity was observed for calretinin (**A**), (100×), Wilms' tumor-1 (WT-1) (**B**), (100×), cytokeratin (CK) 5/6 (**C**), (100×), and vimentin. There was focal staining of epithelial membrane antigen (EMA) and CD10 (non-luminal pattern), whereas the staining for epithelial-cell adhesion molecule (Ep-CAM, BerEP4) (**D**)), (100×), PAX8, Napsin-A, estrogen receptor (ER), renal cell carcinoma antibody (RCC), inhibin, GATA3, and thyroid transcription factor-1 (TTF-1) was negative. The tumor exhibited wild-type expression of p53. Ki-67 proliferative index was 5–10% of cells. The panel of immunohistochemical stains, including the markers supporting mesothelial origin (e.g., calretinin, CK5/6, podoplanin (D2-40), WT1, mesothelin, Hector Battifora mesothelial-1 (HBME-1), or thrombomodulin) and the markers for non-mesothelial neoplasms, is usually helpful in distinguishing mesothelioma from other tumors with similar morphology. It is important to note that if mesothelioma is not considered in the list of differential diagnosis and mesothelial markers are not included, the immunoprofile of mesothelioma can partially overlap with clear-cell adenocarcinoma or other Mullerian-type adenocarcinomas with clear-cell-like features. Mullerian-type adenocarcinomas and mesothelioma are positive for CK7 and EMA. Although negativity for PAX8 and Napsin A is unusual for clear-cell adenocarcinoma, it should be noted that some peritoneal mesotheliomas are positive for PAX8 [8] and Napsin A may be negative in almost 30% of clear-cell adenocarcinomas [16]. WT-1 positivity, as seen in mesothelioma, is characteristic of Mullerian-type serous adenocarcinoma but is unusual for clear-cell adenocarcinoma. Negativity for ER and wild-type p53 pattern is similarly observed in most clear-cell adenocarcinoma and mesothelioma, whereas ER expression is common in serous and endometrioid adenocarcinomas, and abnormal p53 pattern is characteristic of high-grade serous adenocarcinoma [10]. Current recommendations to distinguish mesothelioma from carcinoma is the immunoreactivity for two mesothelial markers and shows negativity for two epithelial carcinoma markers [3]. In this patient, the immunoprofile of calretinin, CK5/6, BerEp4, and PAX8 help exclude clear-cell adenocarcinoma. The location of the tumor in the posterolateral aspect of uterus should also raise the differential diagnosis of rare tumors with mesonephric-related origin, mesonephric carcinoma and Wolffian tumor of uterine ligament. The tumors in this group share similar calretinin positivity. Mesonephric carcinoma is immunopositive for PAX8, GATA3, TTF1 and CD10 (luminal pattern), whereas Wolffian tumor is mostly negative with PAX8 and GATA3. Wolffian tumor is also positive for CK7 and sex cord-stromal markers such as inhibin and FOXL2 [17]. This figure shows the immunohistochemical stains that confirm the diagnosis of clear-cell mesothelioma.

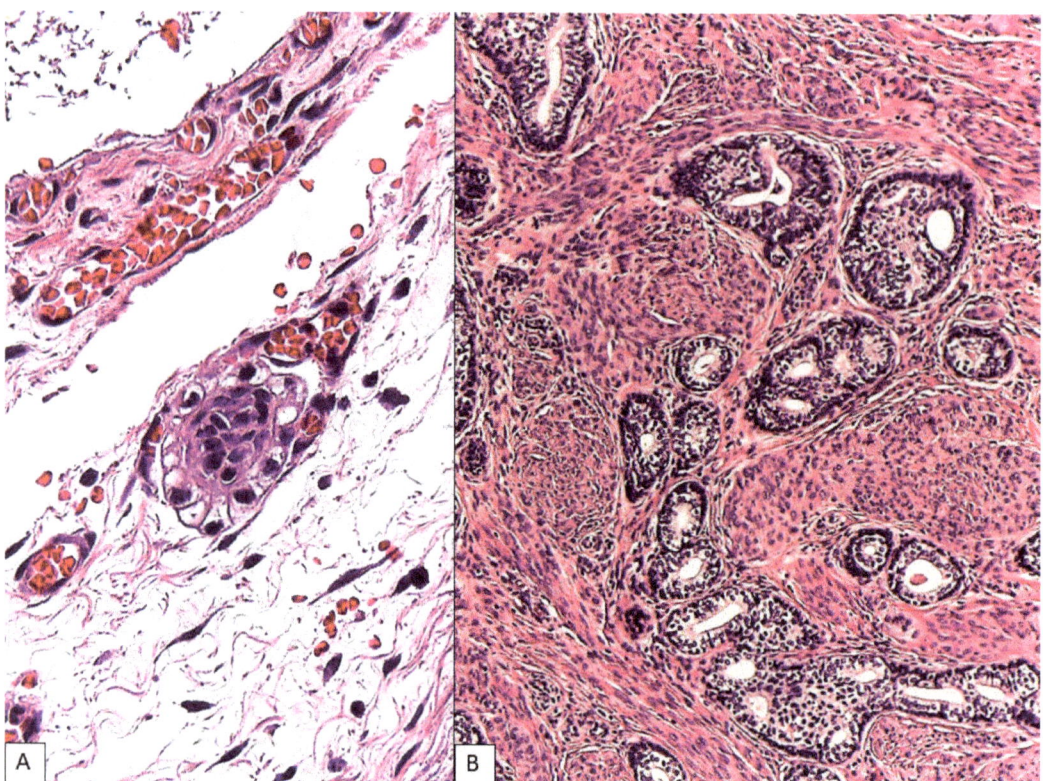

Figure 4. The additional findings in uterus and both adnexa. A cluster of atypical clear cells (less than 0.2 mm) was identified on the surface of left ovary, consistent with metastatic clear-cell mesothelioma (**A**) (H&E, 400×). The cervix showed an incidental adenoid basal carcinoma in the right lateral wall (**B**) (H&E, 100×), measuring 4.5 mm in depth and without lymphovascular involvement (FIGO stage IA2). No neoplastic lesion was seen in the corpus, right ovary, bilateral fallopian tubes, pelvic lymph nodes, omentum, and peritoneal washing cytology. The patient received six cycles of adjuvant chemotherapy and hormonal replacement therapy. She remained well without evidence of disease 12 months after surgery. This figure represents the additional findings after extensive histologic examination of the uterus and both adnexa. A single metastatic focus of the tumor was identified in the contralateral ovarian surface (**A**). In general, localized mesothelioma appears to have a more favorable clinical course than diffuse mesothelioma [6,18]. The prognosis of peritoneal mesothelioma could not be predicted by histomorphology alone, although deciduoid morphology or nuclear grade 3 has been reported to be an independent unfavorable prognostic predictor [2]. Based on NCCN guidelines 2022, epithelioid subtype, Ki-67 index ≤ 9%, peritoneal cancer index of 17 or less, absence of lymph node involvement, and complete cytoreduction are favorable prognostic features [7]. More recently, a novel VHL gene mutation has been reported in peritoneal clear-cell mesothelioma with an indolent clinical behavior [5]. Given the rarity of this entity, the clinical course, prognostic predictors, pathogenesis, and molecular profiles remain to be clarified. This patient had co-existing adenoid basal carcinoma of the uterine cervix (**B**). In a recent series of 18 women with localized peritoneal mesothelioma, a history of other cancers (breast, endometrial, and ovarian) was found in 4 of 13 cases (31%) with available data [6]. Family history available in 11 patients also noted the presence of cancer in their family members in all cases, 82% of which were first-degree relatives. In women with peritoneal mesothelioma, the presence of another tumor should also be monitored [2,6]. In conclusion, clear-cell mesothelioma represents a diagnostic challenge for pathologists. Recognition of this entity, albeit rare, is important as the diagnosis may significantly affect the management considerations.

Author Contributions: T.P. and S.K.: Conceptualization, manuscript writing, pathologic evaluation, final approval; K.S. (Kanokkan Saipattranusorn) and K.S. (Kornkanok Sukpan): reviewing pathologic findings, final approval; P.S.: clinical management, final approval. All authors have read and agreed to the published version of the manuscript.

Funding: This research received no external funding.

Institutional Review Board Statement: The study was conducted in accordance with the Declaration of Helsinki, and approved by the Ethics Committee of Faculty of Medicine, Chiang Mai University (protocol code PAT-2565-09347and date of approval 17 January 2023).

Informed Consent Statement: Written informed consent has been obtained from the patient to publish this paper.

Data Availability Statement: The data of this report are available from the corresponding authors upon request.

Conflicts of Interest: The authors declare no conflict of interest.

References

1. Pavlisko, E.N.; Liu, B.; Green, C.; Sporn, T.A.; Roggli, V.L. Malignant Diffuse Mesothelioma in Women: A Study of 354 Cases. *Am. J. Surg. Pathol.* **2020**, *44*, 293–304. [CrossRef] [PubMed]
2. Malpica, A.; Euscher, E.D.; Marques-Piubelli, M.L.; Ferrufino-Schmidt, M.C.; Miranda, R.N.; Sams, R.; Royal, R.E.; Raghav, K.P.S.; Fournier, K.F.; Ramalingam, P. Malignant Mesothelioma of the Peritoneum in Women: A Clinicopathologic Study of 164 Cases. *Am. J. Surg. Pathol.* **2021**, *45*, 45–58. [CrossRef] [PubMed]
3. Husain, A.N.; Colby, T.V.; Ordonez, N.G.; Allen, T.C.; Attanoos, R.L.; Beasley, M.B.; Butnor, K.J.; Chirieac, L.R.; Churg, A.M.; Dacic, S.; et al. Guidelines for Pathologic Diagnosis of Malignant Mesothelioma 2017 Update of the Consensus Statement from the International Mesothelioma Interest Group. *Arch. Pathol. Lab. Med.* **2018**, *142*, 89–108. [CrossRef] [PubMed]
4. Chapel, D.B.; Schulte, J.J.; Absenger, G.; Attanoos, R.; Brcic, L.; Butnor, K.J.; Chirieac, L.; Churg, A.; Galateau-Salle, F.; Hiroshima, K.; et al. Malignant peritoneal mesothelioma: Prognostic significance of clinical and pathologic parameters and validation of a nuclear-grading system in a multi-institutional series of 225 cases. *Mod. Pathol.* **2021**, *34*, 380–395. [CrossRef] [PubMed]
5. Smith-Hannah, A.; Naous, R. Primary peritoneal epithelioid mesothelioma of clear cell type with a novel VHL gene mutation: A case report. *Hum. Pathol.* **2019**, *83*, 199–203. [CrossRef] [PubMed]
6. Malpica, A.; Euscher, E.D.; Marques-Piubelli, M.L.; Miranda, R.N.; Raghav, K.P.; Fournier, K.F.; Ramalingam, P. Localized Malignant Peritoneal Mesothelioma (LMPeM) in Women: A Clinicopathologic Study of 18 Cases. *Am. J. Surg. Pathol.* **2022**, *46*, 1352–1363. [CrossRef] [PubMed]
7. Singhi, A.D.; Krasinskas, A.M.; Choudry, H.A.; Bartlett, D.L.; Pingpank, J.F.; Zeh, H.J.; Luvison, A.; Fuhrer, K.; Bahary, N.; Seethala, R.R.; et al. The prognostic significance of BAP1, NF2, and CDKN2A in malignant peritoneal mesothelioma. *Mod. Pathol.* **2016**, *29*, 14–24. [CrossRef] [PubMed]
8. National Comprehensive Cancer Network Mesothelioma: Peritoneal (Version:1.2023). Available online: https://www.nccn.org/professionals/physician_gls/pdf/meso_peritoneal.pdf (accessed on 21 February 2023).
9. National Comprehensive Cancer Network. Mesothelioma: Pleural (Version: 1.2023). Available online: https://www.nccn.org/professionals/physician_gls/pdf/meso_pleural.pdf (accessed on 21 February 2023).
10. Centers for Disease Control and Prevention. Incidence of Malignant Mesothelioma, 1999–2018. Available online: https://www.cdc.gov/cancer/uscs/about/data-briefs/no27-incidence-malignant-mesothelioma-1999-2018.htm (accessed on 21 February 2023).
11. Mao, W.; Zhang, X.; Guo, Z.; Gao, Z.; Pass, H.I.; Yang, H.; Carbone, M. Association of Asbestos Exposure with Malignant Mesothelioma Incidence in Eastern China. *JAMA Oncol.* **2017**, *3*, 562–564. [CrossRef] [PubMed]
12. Sugarbaker, P.H.; Welch, L.S.; Mohamed, F.; Glehen, O. A review of peritoneal mesothelioma at the Washington Cancer Institute. *Surg. Oncol. Clin. N. Am.* **2003**, *12*, 605–621. [CrossRef] [PubMed]
13. Zhuo, M.; Zheng, Q.; Chi, Y.; Jia, B.; Zhao, J.; Wu, M.; An, T.; Wang, Y.; Li, J.; Zhao, X.; et al. Survival analysis via nomogram of surgical patients with malignant pleural mesothelioma in the Surveillance, Epidemiology, and End Results database. *Thorac. Cancer* **2019**, *10*, 1193–1202. [CrossRef] [PubMed]
14. Chapel, D.B.; Hornick, J.L.; Barlow, J.; Bueno, R.; Sholl, L.M. Clinical and molecular validation of BAP1, MTAP, P53, and Merlin immunohistochemistry in diagnosis of pleural mesothelioma. *Mod. Pathol.* **2022**, *35*, 1383–1397. [CrossRef] [PubMed]
15. Panou, V.; Gadiraju, M.; Wolin, A.; Weipert, C.M.; Skarda, E.; Husain, A.N.; Patel, J.D.; Rose, B.; Zhang, S.R.; Weatherly, M.; et al. Frequency of Germline Mutations in Cancer Susceptibility Genes in Malignant Mesothelioma. *J. Clin. Oncol* **2018**, *36*, 2863–2871. [CrossRef] [PubMed]
16. Weidemann, S.; Bohle, J.L.; Contreras, H.; Luebke, A.M.; Kluth, M.; Buscheck, F.; Hube-Magg, C.; Hoflmayer, D.; Moller, K.; Fraune, C.; et al. Napsin A Expression in Human Tumors and Normal Tissues. *Pathol. Oncol. Res.* **2021**, *27*, 613099. [CrossRef] [PubMed]

17. Gilk, B. *WHO Classification of Femal Genital Tumours*, 5th ed.; International Agency for Research on Cancer (IARC): Lyon, France, 2020.
18. Marchevsky, A.M.; Khoor, A.; Walts, A.E.; Nicholson, A.G.; Zhang, Y.Z.; Roggli, V.; Carney, J.; Roden, A.C.; Tazelaar, H.D.; Larsen, B.T.; et al. Localized malignant mesothelioma, an unusual and poorly characterized neoplasm of serosal origin: Best current evidence from the literature and the International Mesothelioma Panel. *Mod. Pathol.* **2020**, *33*, 281–296. [CrossRef] [PubMed]

Disclaimer/Publisher's Note: The statements, opinions and data contained in all publications are solely those of the individual author(s) and contributor(s) and not of MDPI and/or the editor(s). MDPI and/or the editor(s) disclaim responsibility for any injury to people or property resulting from any ideas, methods, instructions or products referred to in the content.

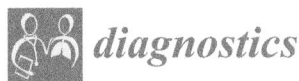

Article

Identifying ITGB2 as a Potential Prognostic Biomarker in Ovarian Cancer

Chanyuan Li [1,2,†], Ting Deng [2,†], Junya Cao [2], Yun Zhou [2], Xiaolin Luo [2], Yanling Feng [2], He Huang [2,*] and Jihong Liu [1,2,*]

1. Cancer Center, The Fifth Affiliated Hospital of Sun Yat-sen University, Zhuhai 519000, China
2. Department of Gynecologic Oncology, State Key Laboratory of Oncology in South China, Collaborative Innovation Center for Cancer Medicine, Sun Yat-sen University, Guangzhou 510060, China
* Correspondence: huangh@sysucc.org.cn (H.H.); liujih@mail.sysu.edu.cn (J.L.)
† These authors contributed equally to this work.

Abstract: Epithelial ovarian cancer is by far the most lethal gynecological malignancy. The exploration of promising immunomarkers to predict prognosis in ovarian cancer patients remains challenging. In our research, we carried out an integrated bioinformatic analysis of genome expressions and their immune characteristics in the ovarian cancer microenvironment with validation in different experiments. We filtrated 332 differentially expressed genes with 10 upregulated hub genes from the Gene Expression Omnibus database. These genes were closely related to ovarian tumorigenesis. Subsequently, the survival and immune infiltration analysis demonstrated that the upregulation of five candidate genes, ITGB2, VEGFA, CLDN4, OCLN, and SPP1, were correlated with an unfavorable clinical outcome and increased immune cell infiltration in ovarian cancer. Of these genes, ITGB2 tended to be the gene most correlated with various immune cell infiltrations and had a strong correlation with significant M2 macrophages infiltration (r = 0.707, $p = 4.71 \times 10^{-39}$), while it had a moderate correlation with CD4+/CD8+ T cells and B cells. This characteristic explains why the high expression of ITGB2 was accompanied by immune activation but did not reverse carcinogenesis. Additionally, we confirmed that ITGB2 was over-expressed in ovarian cancer tissues and was mainly located in cytoplasm, detected by Western blotting and the immunohistochemical method. In summary, ITGB2 may serve as a prognostic immunomarker for ovarian cancer patients.

Keywords: ITGB2; ovarian cancer; prognostic immunomarker

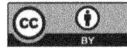

1. Introduction

EOC (Epithelial ovarian cancer) is an aggressive gynecological malignancy with high relapse and mortality rates due to the limited early detection tactics and the absence of effectiveness of existing chemo- and immunotherapies. Thus, it is essential to ascertain alternative diagnostic biomarkers and potential novel targets for ovarian cancer therapy [1,2].

Immuno-oncology has been introduced to the combined treatment of some intractable, advanced malignancies for over a decade, including ovarian cancer patients. The evolution of several immune-based therapies has contributed to effective antitumor responses by regulating the host immune system, including through molecular therapy, cellular therapy in the form of vaccines, CAR-T (Chimeric antigen receptor T-Cell) therapy, and immunomodulator therapy as an immune checkpoint blockade [3,4]. Some clinical trials have incorporated ICIs (immune checkpoint inhibitors) into conventional, platinum-based chemotherapy regimens in serous ovarian cancer patients in combination with cytoreductive surgery, with the aim of reducing the patients' pain and prolonging their survival time [5,6]. Unfortunately, only a minority of patients could benefit from the immune checkpoint blockade treatments through the application of inhibitors of PD-1 (programmed cell death protein 1), such as Sintilimab and Pembrolizumab, and CTLA-4 (cytotoxic T-lymphocyte associated protein 4): Lpilimumab [7–9]. Therefore, novel and effective biomarkers to predict and assess the responses to immunotherapy in serous ovarian cancer are required. Additionally, several studies have reported that an effective antitumor response of immune infiltration would be beneficial to the ICIs' efficacy in patients, and the prognosis of patients particularly depends on the immune infiltration and the epigenetic mutation load of immune cells in the tumor microenvironment [10,11]. Thus, our study intended to demonstrate the possible association between genome expression and tumor-immune interactions in ovarian cancer.

Here, we performed a comprehensive bioinformatic analysis of ITGB2 (integrin beta-2) and its immune-related characteristics in ovarian tumorigenesis. We first found that several genes, including ITGB2, were highly upregulated in serous ovarian cancer samples. Subsequently, the gene and protein interactions with ITGB2 were identified via Metascape and STRING databases, and the high expression of ITGB2 could significantly affect the clinical outcome for patients with serous ovarian cancer. Finally, the TIMER (tumor immune estimation resource) database was employed to evaluate the interactions between ITGB2 and the immune infiltration in the TME (tumor microenvironment). The findings implied that upregulated ITGB2 is particularly related to the infiltration of M2 macrophages. In summary, this study revealed that ITGB2 might function as a prognostic biomarker in ovarian cancer and might lay the groundwork for the landscape of immuno-therapy strategies in advanced serous ovarian cancer.

2. Materials and Methods

2.1. Microarray Data

We obtained the serous-ovarian-cancer-related gene expression datasets and matched non-ovarian cancer sample datasets from the database GEO (gene expression omnibus): https://www.ncbi.nlm.nih.gov/geo/ (accessed on 20 September 2022). The expression profiles selected were GSE36668 and GSE66957.

2.2. DEGs (Differentially Expressed Genes) Identification

We conducted a DEGs analysis between serous ovarian cancers and non-ovarian tumor tissues through the online tool GEO2R via the limma package in the 3.2.3 version R software from https://www.ncbi.nlm.nih.gov/geo/geo2r/ (accessed on 20 September 2022). Genes in the profiles which satisfied the standards of a $|logFC| \geq 2.0$ and an adjusted p value < 0.05 would be confirmed as DEGs. Furthermore, the upregulated differential genes we defined as logFC > 2, and the logFC of downregulated genes was <−2. A Venn diagram analysis was also utilized to probe the intersection of the selected DEGs from http://bioinformatics.psb.ugent.be/webtools/Venn/ (accessed on 20 September 2022).

2.3. Pathway Enrichment and Functional Analysis of the DEGs

Biological function was visualized through a web-based toolkit, Metascape, GO (Gene ontology) enrichment pathways, and KEGG (Kyoto encyclopedia of genes and genomes) -enriched pathways of the genes. Standards included a p-value < 0.01 and minimum > 3. A minimum enrichment factor count of 1.5 would be viewed as statistically significant terms and assembled into clusters on the basis of their similar membership. Then, the immune-associated pathways for ITGB2 would be identified using the Genecards platform: https://www.genecards.org (accessed on 20 September 2022) and the WikiPathways module, and a Reactome pathway analysis was performed.

2.4. Hub Genes Identification

The network PPI (protein–protein interaction) was formulated using the toolkit Cytoscape (version 3.7.1) by screening out the nodes with a composite score > 0.4 (STRING: https://cn.string-db.org (accessed on 20 September 2022). The top 10 genes in the midst of PPI were elicited via the cytoHubba plug-in using the degree algorithm, and a degree score > 38 was selected as a hub gene in our study.

2.5. Hub Genes Prognosis Analysis

The KM (Kaplan–Meier) plotter online toolkit: http://kmplot.com/analysis/ (accessed on 25 September 2022) was utilized to acquire the survival and corresponding clinical information with the criteria: median; hazards ratio: yes; 95% CI (confidence interval): Yes. The hub genes' expression and the particular correlation between the differential genes and various classical surface markers of the infiltrating immune cells were verified using the online platform GEPIA (gene expression profiling interactive analysis): http://gepia.cancer-pku.cn/index.html (accessed on 25 September 2022). Results with an adjusted HR (hazard ratio), a 95% CI, and a log-rank p-value were needed.

2.6. Key Genes Immune Infiltration Analysis

To determine the particular correlation between the prognosis-correlated hub DEGs and a variety of tumor-infiltrating immune cells, we utilized toolkits through the appropriate functional modules: EPIC (estimate the proportion of immune and cancer cells): https://gfellerlab.shinyapps.io/EPIC_1-1/ (accessed on 25 September 2022) and the 2.0 version of the TIMER (tumor immune estimation resource 2.0) database from http://timer.cistrome.org (accessed on 25 September 2022).

2.7. Immunofluorescence

PDC3 (patient-derived ovarian cancer cell) was obtained from Tao Zhu, Professor of The Cancer Hospital of the University of Chinese Academy of Sciences. The PDC3 cell we received was cultured in DMEM/F12 (Dulbecco's modified eagle medium/nutrient mixture12) medium containing 10–15% FBS (Fetal bovine serum) and 1% non-essential amino acid, while the IOSE80 cell (normal ovarian epithelial cell) was cultured in 1640 medium. Both cells were cultured at 37 °C with a 5% CO_2 in a thermostatic incubator. PDC3 and IOSE80 were then incubated with a ITGB2 primary antibody for 2–4 h at 37 °C, followed by an incubation with secondary antibody Alexa Fluor 594 conjugates at 25 °C for 1–2 h. Subsequently, the nucleus and lysosome were stained with Hoechst 33342 a and lysosome-staining kit, respectively, for 10–15 min at room temperature prior to their observation under a confocal microscope (Nikon, A1 HD25, Tokyo, Japan).

2.8. Western Blot

Cell lysates were first obtained by scraping the cultured PDC3 and IOSE80, which were then lysed with a cocktail of protease inhibitors in a RIPA (radioimmunoprecipitation assay) lysis buffer on an ice box (4 °C). Next, the boiled proteins were separated through SDS-PAGE (sodium dodecyl sulphate-polyacrylamide gel electrophoresis) and blocked in PBST (phosphate buffer solution with tween) containing 5% nonfat dried milk. This was followed by incubation with an anti-ITGB2 rabbit monoclonal antibody at 4 °C for 12 h overnight, and a HRP (horseradish peroxidase)-coupled secondary antibody for 2 h. Finally, the target protein bands were detected using a protein imaging system (GE ImageQuant800, Fairfield, CT, USA).

2.9. Immunohistochemistry Analysis

The tumor tissues of 8 serous ovarian cancer patients and 8 non-ovarian tumor controls were collected. Paraffin-embedded tissue sections were cut continuously at 4–5 mm from the tissues and then dewaxed. Next, the antigen was retrieved through the application of a citrate buffer. The tissue slides were then incubated with ITGB2 (Absin, Shanghai, China) primary antibodies overnight or for 12 h at 4 °C. After the 2 h incubation with the secondary antibodies, an ABC (Avidin-biotin complex) Substrate System (Servicebio, Wuhan, China) was applied on the slides for the coloration reaction and with HE (hematoxylin) for counterstaining. Images of the slides and staining were eventually acquired on an Olympus VS200 microscope at 20× magnification. All the quantifications were performed with ImageJ, using IHC (immunohistochemistry) profiler plugins. Positive signals in the epithelial tissue were selected for analysis.

2.10. QRT-PCR (Quantitative, Real Time-Polymerase Chain Reaction)

The total RNA (ribonucleic acid) of the PDC3 and IOSE80 cells was isolated according to the standard procedure with the reagent kit (Vazyme, Nanjing, China) FastPure cell-Tissue Total RNA Isolation Kit V2. The primer sequence of ITGB2 was F5′ ATGTAAGTG-GCCGTCCTTGG 3′, R5′ GGAAGCCGTCACTTTGAGGA 3′. All qPCR experiments were performed by employing the reagent kit (Vazyme, Nanjing, China) HiScript II One Step qRT-PCR SYBR Green Kit and the software Light Cycler96 (Roche, Basel, Switzerland). At least three replicates were used to obtain each average Ct (cycle threshold) value.

2.11. Statistics Analysis

We utilized GraphPad Prism 9.0 to conduct a statistical analysis between the serous ovarian cancer group and the matched non-ovarian tumor group. For parametric data, a two-tailed, unpaired Student's t test was utilized to determine the statistical significance between the two groups. With the data not applicable to a normal distribution, we turned to the nonparametric test, and the Mann–Whitney U test was used to analyze the statistical differences between the groups with the exact method.

3. Results

3.1. DEGs Identification

In this research, we first selected two expression profiles from the GEO database for the subsequent analysis: GSE66957 and GSE36668. The GSE66957 profile consisted of 57 epithelial ovarian cancer tissues and 12 non-tumor tissues, while the GSE36668 encompassed four epithelial ovarian cancer tissues and four matched, non-tumor tissue samples. A volcano plot analysis identified significantly differentially expressed genes in the two datasets, with a standard of p value < 0.05 and $|logFC| \geq 2$ (Figure 1a,b). In total, 1393 DEGs were screened out from the GSE36668. Among these, 732 genes were upregulated and 661 genes were downregulated significantly in serous ovarian cancer tissues. In the GSE66957 profile, 2578 DEGs were screened out, with 1852 upregulated genes and 726 downregulated genes in serous ovarian cancer tissues. All the DEGs were filtered by comparing the epithelial ovarian cancer tissues to the non-ovarian tumor groups. A Venn analysis was then employed to acquire the intersection of these differential genes (Figure 1c,d). Overall, 332 DEGs, including 301 upregulated genes and 31 downregulated genes, were discovered, and the expression heatmap of the genes showed that the over- or under-expression of these DEGs was highly correlated with serous ovarian cancer (Figure 1e,f).

3.2. Analysis of Gene Function and Pathway Enrichment

As we discovered 332 DEGs related to serous ovarian cancer, a series of analyses based on gene annotation and pathway enrichment on the above 332 DEGs were conducted via Metascape. Analyses were conducted for the sake of exploring the potential biological function of the differential genes. Results suggested that these DEGs were majorly enriched in the regulation of cell adhesion, cell–cell adhesion, cell junction organization, the integrin-mediated signaling pathway, and extracellular matrix organization (Figure 2a,b). The details of the annotation and enrichment information of the 332 DEGs were presented in Table S1. In conclusion, the serous-ovarian-cancer-related DEGs we identified may play a pivotal role in cell communications and transitions.

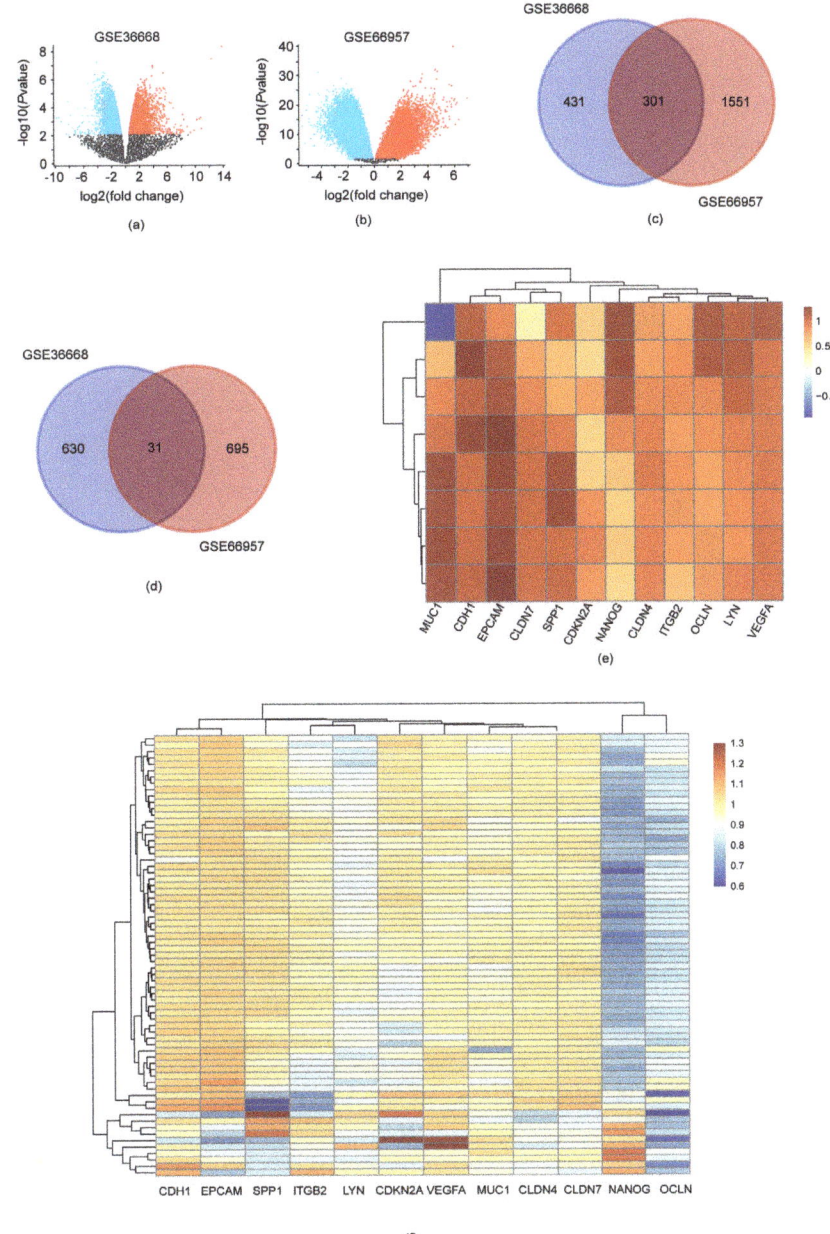

Figure 1. DEGs of two expression profiles. (**a**) Differentially expressed genes in profile GSE36668, identified with volcano plot; (**b**) Differentially expressed genes in profile GSE66957, identified with volcano plot. (The blue dots indicate downregulated genes in serous ovarian cancer patients, and red dots indicate upregulated genes in serous ovarian cancer patients); (**c**) Venn analysis of the up-regulated genes in two profiles; (**d**) Venn analysis of the down-regulated genes in two profiles; (**e**) Heatmap representing several selected DEGs between ovarian cancer and control groups in GSE36668 profile (one sample per raw); (**f**) Heatmap representing several selected DEGs between ovarian cancer and control group in GSE66957 profile (one sample per raw).

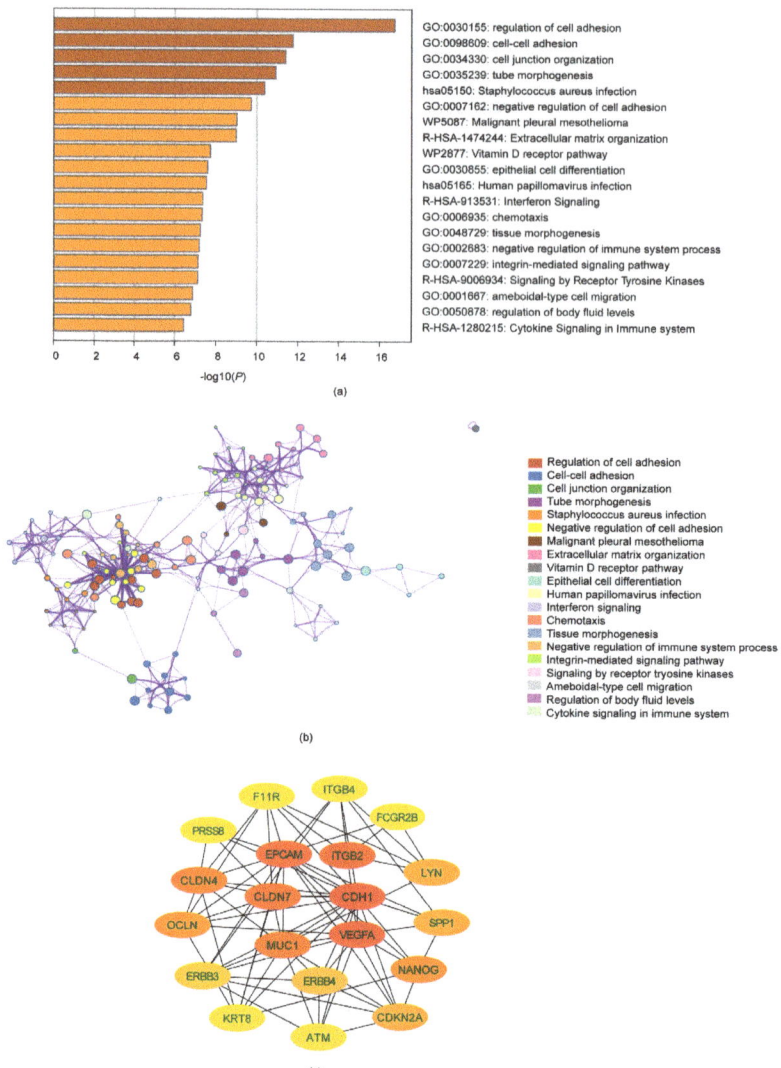

Figure 2. Enrichment analysis of the DEGs. (**a**) Top 20 functional enrichment results from the enrichment analyses of DEGs screened by Metascape; (**b**) The visualization of top 20 enriched terms of DEGs; each specific color is indicated with a cluster ID; (**c**) Hub genes' interaction network constructed by Cytoscape. The score is exhibited in the color orange: a darker color usually indicates a higher score in this network.

3.3. Identification of Ten Hub Genes through PPI

The hub genes of the DEGs were further selected using STRING and Cytoscape. The DEGs' interactional proteins were first predicted via the STRING database, and then the densest connection modes were analyzed using the Cytoscape platform. The top ten genes in the PPI network were CDH1 (Cadherin 1), EPCAM (epithelial cell adhesion molecule), ITGB2, CLDN7 (Claudin7), VEGFA (vascular endothelial growth factor A), MUC1 (polymorphic epithelial mucin1), CLDN4 (Claudin4), NANOG (Nanog homeobox), OCLN (Occludin), CDKN2A (Cyclin-dependent kinase inhibitor 2A), LYN (LYN proto-oncogene, Src family tyrosine kinase), and SPP1 (secreted phosphoprotein 1) (Table S2).

The hub genes' expression differences between the serous ovarian cancer tissues and the non-ovarian tumor tissues in the two profiles a shown in Figure 1e,f). Among these, DH1, VEGFA, EPCAM, ITGB2, and CLDN7 had the highest correlation scores with serous ovarian cancer.

3.4. ITGB2, VEGFA, CLDN4, OCLN, and SPP1 Were Correlated with Poor Prognosis in Serous Ovarian Cancer Patients

To seek the candidate biomarkers with prognostic potency, we performed an analysis of the capacity of the ten candidate genes to predict the prognosis of patients via the online Kaplan–Meier plotter platform. Interestingly, we discovered that the PFS (progression-free survival) was significantly reduced in ovarian cancer patients when the expression level of the related genes was high ($p < 0.05$), as were the related hub genes, including ITGB2 (HR = 1.24, $p = 0.0027$), VEGFA (HR = 1.38, $p = 1.8 \times 10^{-5}$), CLDN4 (HR = 1.22, $p = 0.0047$), OCLN (HR = 1.38, $p = 9.1 \times 10^{-6}$), and SPP1 (HR = 1.38, $p = 7.7 \times 10^{-7}$). This indicates that the active transcription of these genes might cause risks in tumorigenesis. Therefore, the five genes might have the potential to be alternative prognostic biomarkers for serous ovarian cancer patients (Figure 3a). We additionally employed the GEPIA database to confirm the expression of these candidates in serous ovarian cancer tissues and nonovarian tumor tissues, indicating that the over-expression of genes was positive relative to serous ovarian cancer ($p < 0.05$). The differential expression of five key genes in ovarian tumors and non-ovarian tumor tissues through the GEPIA dataset are shown in Figure 3b,c. The differential expression in serous ovarian cancer tissues and non-ovarian cancer tissues may also explain the trend we observed from the GEO database. These results therefore clearly demonstrated that the expression of ITGB2, VEGFA, CLDN4, OCLN, and SPP1 were significantly correlated with poorer clinical outcomes in serous ovarian cancer.

3.5. ITGB2 Was Associated with TAM (Tumor-Associated Macrophage) Infiltration in Serous Ovarian Cancer

Previous studies [12–14] reported that the survival rate could be independently evaluated by the frequency of various tumor-infiltrating lymphocytes in patients bearing a solid malignant tumor as well as a hematologic tumor. We explored the underlying connection between the five candidate genes and their characteristic immune infiltration in a tumor-immune microenvironment via the TIMER and EPIC databases. First, we used the EPIC database to draw up the major immune cell types in two profiles. Interestingly, the results showed that the immune microenvironment appeared to be characterized by a dilemma between immune activation and immune suppression (Figure S1). We next assessed the particular association between five genes and then a variety of infiltrating immune cells in serous ovarian cancer, such as CD4+/CD8+ T cells, B cells, and macrophages. Importantly, we found that ITGB2 in the serous ovarian cancer microenvironment was positively correlated with immune infiltration compared to the other four prognosis-related genes, and it had a strong correlation with the infiltration of macrophages, such as macrophages ($r = 0.3107$, $p = 3.17 \times 10^{-7}$), M0 macrophages ($r = 0.157$, $p = 1.32 \times 10^{-2}$), M1 macrophages ($r = 0.3053$, $p = 1.02 \times 10^{-8}$), and M2 macrophages ($r = 0.707$, $p = 4.71 \times 10^{-39}$), in serous ovarian cancer, while it had a moderate correlation with CD4+/CD8+ T cells (cluster of differentiation 4 + Tregs/cluster of differentiation 8 + Tregs) (Table S3). This feature explains why immune activation and suppression coexist in the ovarian cancer microenvironment (Figure 4a,b). In addition, we also probed into the relationship between the five key genes and a variety of the immune cell-surface genes of TAMs, M0 macrophages, M1 macrophages, and M2 macrophages via the GEPIA database, which indicated a positive correlation between ITGB2 expression and most of the genetic surface markers in macrophages, M1 macrophages, M2 macrophages, and TAMs (Table S4). However, there was no significant correlation between the other four genes with macrophage infiltration. For this reason, we selected ITGB2 as the top candidate prognostic biomarker and focused on the role of ITGB2 in the serous ovarian cancer microenvironment. Additionally, ITGB2 has the potential to be an indicator of pan-cancer immune infiltration (Figure 4c). The above findings in our study implicate that ITGB2 may affect the prognosis of serous ovarian cancer patients, possibly through remodeling the tumor immune microenvironment.

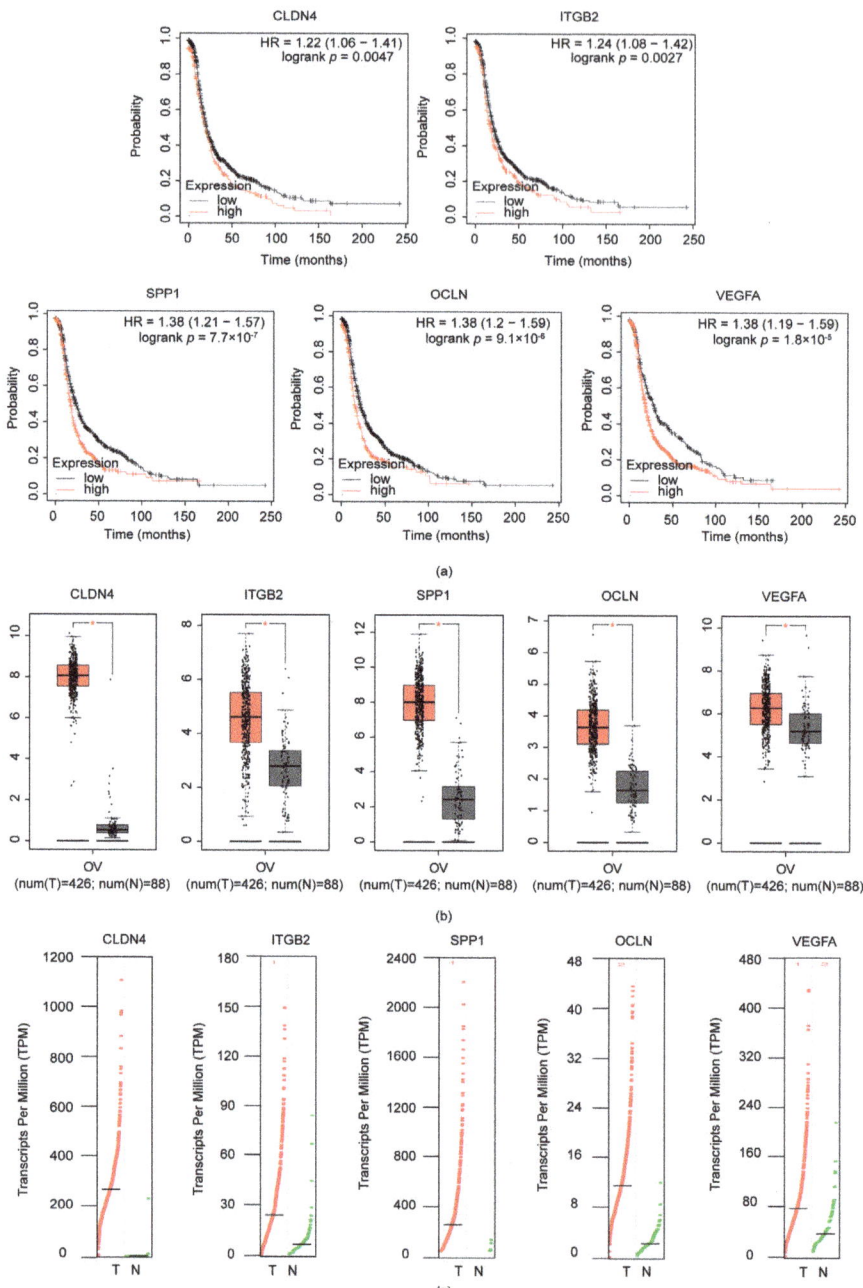

Figure 3. Potential expression of prognostic hub genes in ovarian cancer. (**a**) ITGB2, VEGFA, CLDN4, OCLN, and SPP1 were correlated with unfavorable progression free survival for serous ovarian cancer patients; (**b**,**c**) Expression of ITGB2, VEGFA, CLDN4, OCLN, and SPP1 in serous ovarian cancers, compared with non-ovarian tumor tissues (* $p < 0.05$).

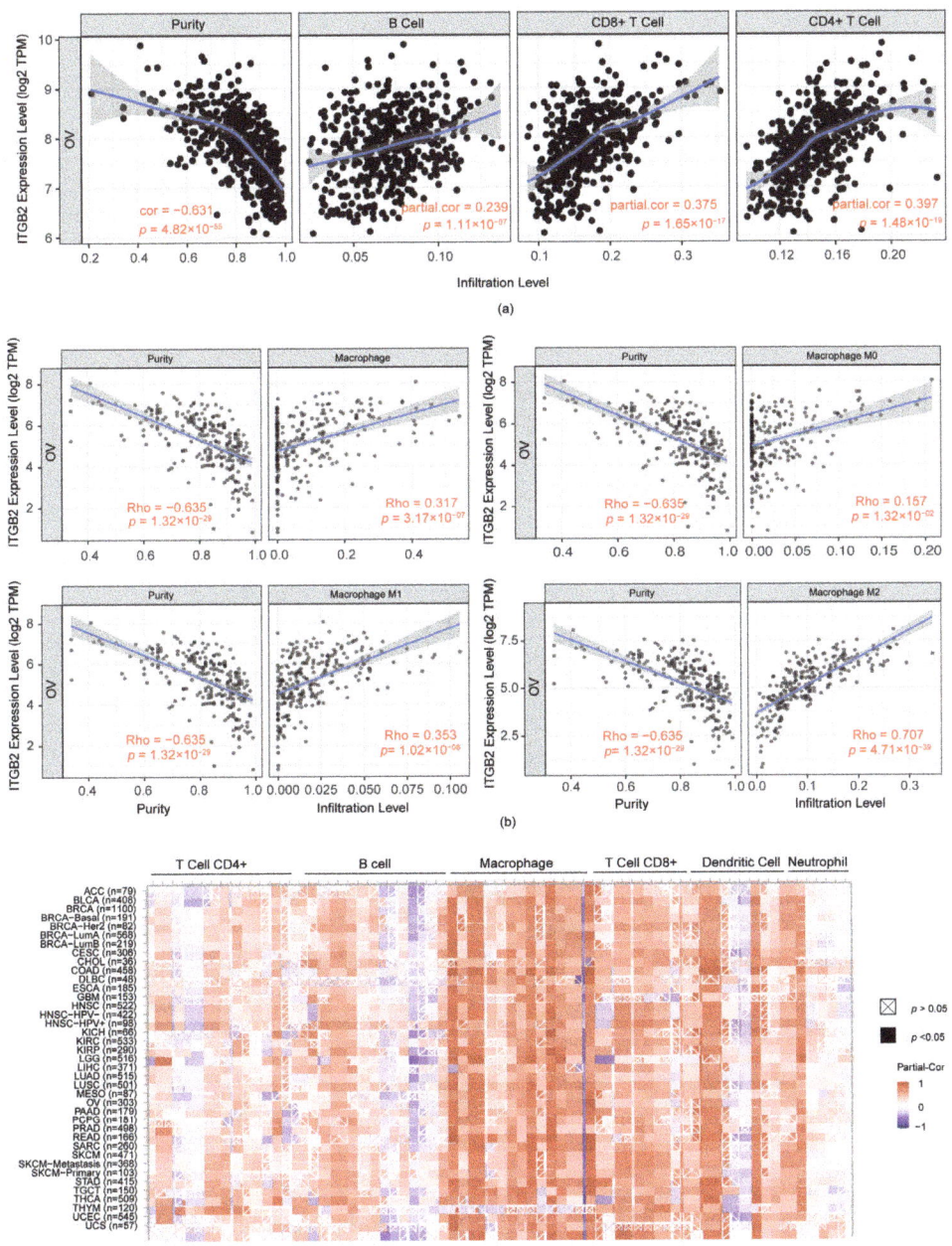

Figure 4. Relevance between ITGB2 expression and infiltration of classical immune cells. (**a**) Relevance between ITGB2 and a variety of infiltrating immune cells (B cells, CD4+/CD8+ T cells); (**b**) Relevance between ITGB2 and macrophages, including: macrophages, M0 macrophages, M1 macrophages, and M2 macrophages; (**c**) Relevance between ITGB2 expression and classical immune cells in other cancer types in patients.

3.6. Validation the Expression of ITGB2 in Serous Ovarian Cancer

Having demonstrated the potential relationship between ITGB2 and the immune infiltration in serous ovarian cancer patients via an integrated bioinformatics analysis, we deduced that this association may also be applicable to serous ovarian cancer patients. Hence, for the sake of verifying the possible correlation between ITGB2 and serous ovarian cancer, we evaluated the expression and cellular localization of ITGB2 in serous ovarian cancer and non-ovarian tumor cells or tissues via a series of experiments. Consistent with the previous findings, the expression of ITGB2 was increased significantly in serous ovarian cancer cells compared to normal ovarian epithelial cells both in protein and mRNA (messenger ribonucleic acid) levels. Results show that the relative expression of ITGB2 mRNA in the patient-derived ovarian cancer cell (PDC3) was 1.625, which was significantly upregulated (p = 0.0304 < 0.05) compared with the expression in the IOSE80 cell (mRNA = 1). (Figure 5b,c). Additionally, ITGB2 was found to be positively expressed (27.27%) in the cytoplasm in serous ovarian cancer cells and tissues (Figure 5a–d) but was almost negative (5.93%) in the normal ovarian epithelial cells and non-tumor tissues, with a significant difference (p < 0.0001) (Figure 5e). This indicates that the upregulation of ITGB2 might play a role in serous ovarian cancer.

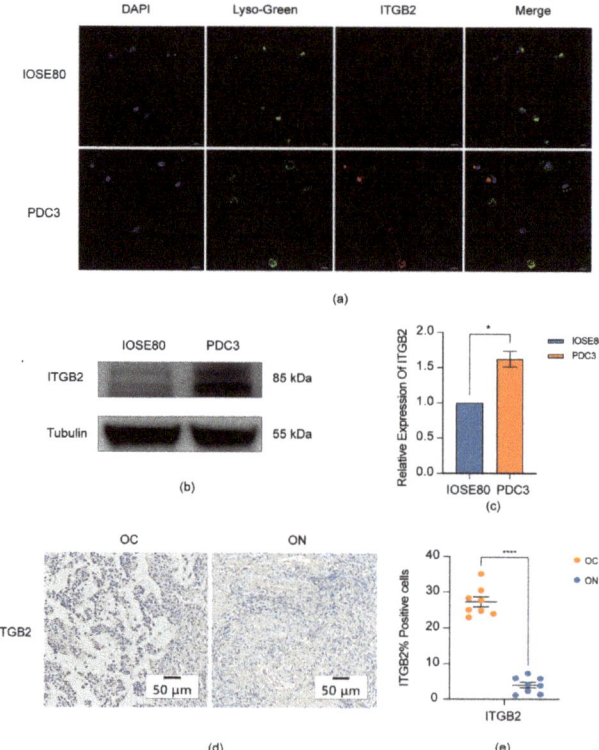

Figure 5. Validation of the expression of ITGB2 in PDC and specimens. (**a**) Location of ITGB2 in two ovarian cancer patient-derived cells via confocal microscopy (red: ITGB2; blue: cell nucleus; green: cell lysosome; scale bar = 20 μm); (**b**) Expression of ITGB2 in IOSE80 and PDC3 cells by Western blotting; (**c**) Detection the relative mRNA expression of ITGB2 via qPCR (* p < 0.05); (**d**) Representative immunohistochemical staining of ITGB2 in serous ovarian cancer tissues and control tissues. (OC: ovarian cancer; ON: matched control ovarian tissues); (**e**) Quantification of ITGB2-positive cells in tumor tissues (**** p < 0.0001, two-tailed, unpaired Student's t test). At least two independent experiments were performed, and the data in the figure are shown as means ± SEM.

3.7. Immune-Associated Pathways for ITGB2

Since the upregulated ITGB2 was connected with the immune infiltration in serous ovarian cancer, we further applied Wikipathways and Reactome analyses for the potential molecular mechanism of ITGB2. The Reactome analysis revealed that ITGB2 was most related to an adaptive and innate immune system in the host. ITGB2 could influence the immunoregulatory crosstalk between a lymphoid and a non-lymphoid cell in the adaptive immune system in host while participating in FCGR (Fc-gamma receptor)-dependent phagocytosis in the innate immune system. The common pathways between the innate and adaptive immune system, including integrin cell-surface interactions, toll-like receptor cascades, neutrophil degranulation, interleukin-4, and interleukin-13 signaling. In addition to, the WikiPathways analysis also showed that the PI3K/Akt/mTOR signaling pathway (phosphatidylinositol 3 kinase-protein kinase b-mammalian target of rapamycin) was the most involved in focal adhesion and the integrin-mediated cell adhesion pathways (Figures S2 and S3). Cause cell adhesion and focal adhesion are associated with the immune system; these results encouraged us to further probe the regulatory effects of ITGB2 on the immune system, and the mechanism of the function might have relevance to the influence of the PI3K/Akt/mTOR signaling pathway.

4. Discussion

Despite tremendous progress in immunotherapy, epithelial ovarian cancer patients remain poorly responsive to it, probably due to immunosuppression and the high heterogeneity. Therefore, to enhance the clinical efficacy of immunotherapy by heating the "cold" ovarian cancer, further studies on new therapies and the molecular mechanisms in the ovarian cancer tumor immune microenvironment remain to be elucidated [15,16].

The tumor microenvironment consists of abundant stromal components, which are composed of various cell types, including the extracellular matrix, fibroblasts, chondrocytes, and mesothelial cells, non-stromal components comprising different immune cells and adipocytes, and microbiota, such as mycoplasma [17,18]. Indubitably, the diverse cellular compositions play a crucial role in the heterogeneity of serous ovarian cancers and induce the initiation, progression, and resistance to the anti-tumor therapy of serous ovarian cancer [19,20]. Macrophages are plastic mononuclear phagocytic cells which can polarize into specific functional phenotypes with the stimulation of some cytokines. TAMs, originating from tissue-resident macrophages, are the most predominant subgroup of immune cells in the ovarian cancer microenvironment. TAMs usually play a pro-tumorigenic role in the tumor microenvironment, functioning to drive tumor proliferation and metastasis [21]. This could polarize into tumoricidal M1 macrophages and tumorigenic M2 macrophages. M2 macrophages commonly predominate in the ovarian cancer environment [22,23]. Thus, it may be crucial to reprogram the TAMs in TME to improve the strong immunosuppression and increase therapeutic effectiveness of ovarian cancer, with the aim of providing a new insight for immunotherapy in ovarian cancer [24,25]. Interestingly, based on the assessments of the TIMER and EPIC databases, we found that the tumor environment comprised CAFs (cancer-associated fibroblasts), CD4+/CD8+ T cells, and macrophages, revealing that the immune microenvironment of ovarian cancer presents a dichotomy between immune activation and suppression. This dynamic characteristic explains why the high expression of ITGB2 is accompanied by the immune activation, but does not reverse carcinogenesis [26]. Across the databases, we also found that ITGB2 has a positive relevance to immune infiltration in a various of cancer types, including ovarian cancer. This study consistently observed that ITGB2 was moderately connected with the CD4+/CD8+ T cell and B cell infiltration, while it was significantly associated with macrophage infiltration. An additional key finding was that the ITGB2 expression was significantly higher in M2 macrophages compared with M0 macrophages and M1 macrophages. This implies that ITGB2 might play a decisive role in regulating TAMs differentiation.

ITGB2, also known as CD18/LFA-1, is a transmembrane cell surface receptor attached to the integrin family. It can encode integrin beta chains and bind to the alpha chains, forming the versatile integrin heterodimers. ITGB2 can be involved in cell adhesion as well as the cell-surface mediated signaling pathway, functioning as hemidesmosomes in the transition and maturation in a various of immune cells and contributing to the interplay between the immune system and the organism, thereby motivating tumorigenesis. [27–29]. Additionally, studies by Grabbe showed that Tregs adhere to DCs (dendritic cells) via ITGB2, leading to an impaired antigen presentation ability and the inhibition of T-cells, revealing the possible mechanism of T cell activation [30]. ITGB2 plays a vital role in in various disorders covering nasopharyngeal carcinoma, NSCLC (non-small cell lung cancer), glioma, breast cancer, and osteosarcoma, and non-tumor diseases, including the SSc (systemic sclerosis) and NEC (necrotizing enterocolitis) of infants [31]. Research by Wang's group [32] demonstrated that the ITGB2/FAK/SOX6 (focal adhesion kinase/SRY-box containing gene 6) pathway was activated to promote metastasis, invasion, and glycolysis in nasopharyngeal carcinoma via phosphorylation and protein interactions, which may offer a novel target for the therapy of nasopharyngeal carcinoma. Additionally, previous research also reported that ITGB2 was upregulated in osteosarcoma, [33] which could drive tumor metastasis via the ITGB2/FAK pathway [34]. Xu [35] reported that the expression of ITGB2 in NSCLC was associated with Treg cells and MDSC (myeloid-derived suppressor cell) infiltration positively. They found that the upregulation of ITGB2 in NSCLC cell lines increased the expression of immune-related proteins, such as N-cadherin, snail, and slug, while decreasing the E-cadherin expression, laying the foundation for further research on immunotherapy. Regarding the non-tumor disorders, studies suggested that the upregulated mRNA expression level of ITGB2 in PBMCs (peripheral blood mononuclear cells) did not associate with disease severity of SSc patients, nor did the status in premature infants with NEC [36,37]. Our results highlight the potential ability of ITGB2 to be a regulator of immune infiltration and a marker of the response to immunotherapy for ovarian cancer patients.

5. Conclusions

Generally, we conducted an integrated bioinformatic analysis of genome expression and immune characteristics in serous ovarian cancer with validation in different experiments. We revealed that the expression of ITGB2, VEGFA, CLDN4, OCLN, and SPP1 were increased in serous ovarian cancer tissues compared with non-ovarian tumor ovarian tissues, and that the upregulation of these genes was associated with immune infiltration and a poor clinical outcome in serous ovarian cancer patients. Additionally, ITGB2 might function as a novel prognostic biomarker for immunotherapy and might work as a biomarker for efficacy prediction, monitoring toxic and adverse effects of immunotherapy, and even to screen the refractory patients suitable for immunotherapy. Furthermore, we identified the specific expression of ITGB2 in both ovarian cancer patient-derived cells and tumor tissues. Thus, this study identified, for the first time, that ITGB2 may act as a novel prognostic immunomarker for ovarian cancer patients.

Supplementary Materials: The following supporting information can be downloaded at: https://www.mdpi.com/article/10.3390/diagnostics13061169/s1, Table S1: Top 20 significantly enriched GO terms and biological functional pathways of DEGs; Table S2: Top ten in network string interactions, ranked by degree method and their *p* value of the progression-free survival analysis; Table S3: Correlation between CLDN4, OCLN, SPP1, and VEGFA expression and the level of immune infiltration; Table S4: Correlation analysis between five hub genes and markers of macrophages in GEPIA; Figure S1: The proportion of immune cells in the GSE36668 and GSE66957 datasets; Figure S2: Integrin-mediated cell adhesion pathway; Figure S3: Focal adhesion: PI3K/Akt/mTOR signaling pathway.

Author Contributions: C.L. and T.D. contributed equally to the study's conceptualization and design. J.C., Y.Z. and X.L. assisted with the study of data and performed bioinformatics analyses. The manuscript was revised with the help of Y.F., H.H. and J.L. The final manuscript was read and approved by all authors. C.L. and T.D. contributed equally to this work. All authors have read and agreed to the published version of the manuscript.

Funding: This research was supported by the National Natural Science Foundation of China (No. 81972443 to J.H. Liu).

Institutional Review Board Statement: This research was approved by the Ethical Committee of the Zhejiang Cancer Hospital (ZRB-2021-242, 2021-7-16).

Informed Consent Statement: Informed consent was obtained from all subjects involved in the study. Written informed consent was obtained from the patients to publish this paper.

Data Availability Statement: The bioinformatics data we used were obtained from online database including GEO, GEPIA, Kaplan–Meier plotter, EPIC, and TIMER2.0.

Conflicts of Interest: The authors declare no conflict of interest.

References

1. Orr, B.; Edwards, R.P. Diagnosis and Treatment of Ovarian Cancer. *Hematol. Oncol. Clin. N. Am.* **2018**, *32*, 943–964. [CrossRef] [PubMed]
2. Paffenholz, S.V.; Salvagno, C.; Ho, Y.J.; Limjoco, M.; Baslan, T.; Tian, S.; Kulick, A.; de Stanchina, E.; Wilkinson, J.E.; Barriga, F.M.; et al. Senescence induction dictates response to chemo- and immunotherapy in preclinical models of ovarian cancer. *Proc. Natl. Acad. Sci. USA* **2022**, *119*, e2117754119. [CrossRef] [PubMed]
3. Yap, T.A.; Parkes, E.E.; Peng, W.; Moyers, J.T.; Curran, M.A.; Tawbi, H.A. Development of Immunotherapy Combination Strategies in Cancer. *Cancer Discov.* **2021**, *11*, 1368–1397. [CrossRef]
4. Del Paggio, J.C. Immunotherapy: Cancer immunotherapy and the value of cure. *Nat. Rev. Clin. Oncol.* **2018**, *15*, 268–270. [CrossRef] [PubMed]
5. Chen, J.; Chen, S.; Dai, X.; Ma, L.; Chen, Y.; Bian, W.; Sun, Y. Exploration of the underlying biological differences and targets in ovarian cancer patients with diverse immunotherapy response. *Front. Immunol.* **2022**, *13*, 1480. [CrossRef]
6. Lee, Y.J.; Woo, H.Y.; Kim, Y.N.; Park, J.; Nam, E.J.; Kim, S.W.; Kim, S.; Kim, Y.T.; Park, E.; Joung, J.G.; et al. Dynamics of the Tumor Immune Microenvironment during Neoadjuvant Chemotherapy of High-Grade Serous Ovarian Cancer. *Cancers* **2022**, *14*, 2308. [CrossRef]
7. Yigit, R.; Massuger, L.F.; Figdor, C.G.; Torensma, R. Ovarian cancer creates a suppressive microenvironment to escape immune elimination. *Gynecol. Oncol.* **2010**, *117*, 366–372. [CrossRef]
8. Ghisoni, E.; Imbimbo, M.; Zimmermann, S.; Valabrega, G. Ovarian Cancer Immunotherapy: Turning up the Heat. *Int. J. Mol. Sci.* **2019**, *20*, 2927. [CrossRef]
9. Odunsi, K. Immunotherapy in ovarian cancer. *Ann. Oncol.* **2017**, *28*, viii1–viii7. [CrossRef]
10. Binnewies, M.; Roberts, E.W.; Kersten, K.; Chan, V.; Fearon, D.F.; Merad, M.; Coussens, L.M.; Gabrilovich, D.I.; Ostrand-Rosenberg, S.; Hedrick, C.C.; et al. Understanding the tumor immune microenvironment (TIME) for effective therapy. *Nat. Med.* **2018**, *24*, 541–550. [CrossRef]
11. Wang, S.; Fu, Y.; Kuerban, K.; Liu, J.; Huang, X.; Pan, D.; Chen, H.; Zhu, Y.; Ye, L. Discoidin domain receptor 1 is a potential target correlated with tumor invasion and immune infiltration in gastric cancer. *Front. Immunol.* **2022**, *13*, 933165. [CrossRef] [PubMed]
12. Zeng, D.; Li, M.; Zhou, R.; Zhang, J.; Sun, H.; Shi, M.; Bin, J.; Liao, Y.; Rao, J.; Liao, W. Tumor Microenvironment Characterization in Gastric Cancer Identifies Prognostic and Immunotherapeutically Relevant Gene Signatures. *Cancer Immunol. Res.* **2019**, *7*, 737–750. [CrossRef] [PubMed]
13. Tobin, J.W.D.; Keane, C.; Mollee, P.; Birch, S.; Gould, C.; Gunawardana, J.; Hoang, T.; Ma, T.; Abro, E.U.; Shanavas, M.; et al. The Tumor Microenvironment Is Independently Prognostic of Conventional and Clinicogenetic Risk Models in Follicular Lymphoma. *Blood* **2017**, *130*, 728. [CrossRef]
14. Cheng, B.; Yu, Q.; Wang, W. Intimate communications within the tumor microenvironment: Stromal factors function as an orchestra. *J. Biomed. Sci.* **2023**, *30*, 1. [CrossRef]
15. Kandalaft, L.E.; Dangaj Laniti, D.; Coukos, G. Immunobiology of high-grade serous ovarian cancer: Lessons for clinical translation. 2022, 22, 640–656. *Nat. Rev. Cancer* **2022**, *22*, 640–656. [CrossRef]
16. Rajtak, A.; Ostrowska-Lesko, M.; Zak, K.; Tarkowski, R.; Kotarski, J.; Okla, K. Integration of local and systemic immunity in ovarian cancer: Implications for immunotherapy. *Front. Immunol.* **2022**, *13*, 1018256. [CrossRef]
17. Zhao, Y.; Mei, S.; Huang, Y.; Chen, J.; Zhang, X.; Zhang, P. Integrative analysis deciphers the heterogeneity of cancer-associated fibroblast and implications on clinical outcomes in ovarian cancers. *Comput. Struct. Biotechnol. J.* **2022**, *20*, 6403–6411. [CrossRef]
18. Siminzar, P.; Tohidkia, M.R.; Eppard, E.; Vahidfar, N.; Tarighatnia, A.; Aghanejad, A. Recent Trends in Diagnostic Biomarkers of Tumor Microenvironment. *Mol. Imaging Biol.* **2022**, 1–19. [CrossRef]
19. Hanahan, D.; Weinberg, R.A. Hallmarks of cancer: The next generation. *Cell* **2011**, *144*, 646–674. [CrossRef]
20. Yang, Y.; Yang, Y.; Yang, J.; Zhao, X.; Wei, X. Tumor Microenvironment in Ovarian Cancer: Function and Therapeutic Strategy. *Front. Cell Dev. Biol.* **2020**, *8*, 758. [CrossRef]
21. Colvin, E.K. Tumor-associated macrophages contribute to tumor progression in ovarian cancer. *Front. Oncol.* **2014**, *4*, 137. [CrossRef] [PubMed]

22. Allavena, P.; Sica, A.; Garlanda, C.; Mantovani, A. The Yin-Yang of tumor-associated macrophages in neoplastic progression and immune surveillance. *Immunol. Rev.* **2008**, *222*, 155–161. [CrossRef] [PubMed]
23. Zanganeh, S.; Spitler, R.; Hutter, G.; Ho, J.Q.; Pauliah, M.; Mahmoudi, M. Tumor-associated macrophages, nanomedicine and imaging: The axis of success in the future of cancer immunotherapy. *Immunotherapy* **2017**, *9*, 819–835. [CrossRef] [PubMed]
24. Truxova, I.; Cibula, D.; Spisek, R.; Fucikova, J. Targeting tumor-associated macrophages for successful immunotherapy of ovarian carcinoma. *J. Immunother. Cancer* **2023**, *11*, e005968. [CrossRef]
25. Lin, Y.; Zhou, X.; Ni, Y.; Zhao, X.; Liang, X. Metabolic reprogramming of the tumor immune microenvironment in ovarian cancer: A novel orientation for immunotherapy. *Front. Immunol.* **2022**, *13*, 1030831. [CrossRef]
26. Xu, H.; Zhang, A.; Han, X.; Li, Y.; Zhang, Z.; Song, L.; Wang, W.; Lou, M. ITGB2 as a prognostic indicator and a predictive marker for immunotherapy in gliomas. *Cancer Immunol. Immunother.* **2022**, *71*, 645–660. [CrossRef]
27. Schittenhelm, L.; Hilkens, C.M.; Morrison, V.L. β2 Integrins As Regulators of Dendritic Cell, Monocyte, and Macrophage Function. *Front. Immunol.* **2017**, *8*, 1866. [CrossRef]
28. Brücher, B.L.D.M.; Jamall, I.S. Cell-Cell Communication in the Tumor Microenvironment, Carcinogenesis, and Anticancer Treatment. *Cell. Physiol. Biochem.* **2014**, *34*, 213–243. [CrossRef]
29. Wei, J.; Huang, X.J.; Huang, Y.; Xiong, M.Y.; Yao, X.Y.; Huang, Z.N.; Li, S.N.; Zhou, W.J.; Fang, D.L.; Deng, D.H.; et al. Key immune-related gene ITGB2 as a prognostic signature for acute myeloid leukemia. *Ann. Transl. Med.* **2021**, *9*, 1386. [CrossRef]
30. Varga, G.; Balkow, S.; Wild, M.K.; Stadtbaeumer, A.; Krummen, M.; Rothoeft, T.; Higuchi, T.; Beissert, S.; Wethmar, K.; Scharffetter-Kochanek, K.; et al. Active MAC-1 (CD11b/CD18) on DCs inhibits full T-cell activation. *Blood* **2006**, *109*, 661–669. [CrossRef]
31. Liu, H.; Wang, J.; Luo, T.; Zhen, Z.; Liu, L.; Zheng, Y.; Zhang, C.; Hu, X. Correlation between ITGB2 expression and clinical characterization of glioma and the prognostic significance of its methylation in low-grade glioma(LGG). *Front. Endocrinol.* **2022**, *13*, 1106120. [CrossRef]
32. Li, J.; Zhang, Z.; Feng, X.; Shen, Z.; Sun, J.; Zhang, X.; Bu, F.; Xu, M.; Tan, C.; Wang, Z. Stanniocalcin-2 promotes cell EMT and glycolysis via activating ITGB2/FAK/SOX6 signaling pathway in nasopharyngeal carcinoma. *Cell Biol. Toxicol.* **2022**, *38*, 259–272. [CrossRef]
33. Benedicto, A.; Marquez, J.; Herrero, A.; Olaso, E.; Kolaczkowska, E.; Arteta, B. Decreased expression of the beta2 integrin on tumor cells is associated with a reduction in liver metastasis of colorectal cancer in mice. *BMC Cancer* **2017**, *17*, 827. [CrossRef] [PubMed]
34. Harburger, D.S.; Calderwood, D.A. Integrin signalling at a glance. *J. Cell Sci.* **2009**, *122*, 1472. [CrossRef]
35. Zu, L.; He, J.; Zhou, N.; Zeng, J.; Zhu, Y.; Tang, Q.; Jin, X.; Zhang, L.; Xu, S. The Profile and Clinical Significance of ITGB2 Expression in Non-Small-Cell Lung Cancer. *J. Clin. Med.* **2022**, *11*, 6421. [CrossRef] [PubMed]
36. George, L.; Menden, H.; Xia, S.; Yu, W.; Holmes, A.; Johnston, J.; Reid, K.J.; Josephson, C.D.; Patel, R.M.; Ahmed, A.; et al. ITGB2 (Integrin beta2) Immunomodulatory Gene Variants in Premature Infants With Necrotizing Enterocolitis. *J. Pediatr. Gastroenterol. Nutr.* **2021**, *72*, e37–e41. [CrossRef]
37. Dashti, N.; Mahmoudi, M.; Gharibdoost, F.; Kavosi, H.; Rezaei, R.; Imeni, V.; Jamshidi, A.; Aslani, S.; Mostafaei, S.; Vodjgani, M. Evaluation of ITGB2 (CD18) and SELL (CD62L) genes expression and methylation of ITGB2 promoter region in patients with systemic sclerosis. *Rheumatol. Int.* **2018**, *38*, 489–498. [CrossRef]

Disclaimer/Publisher's Note: The statements, opinions and data contained in all publications are solely those of the individual author(s) and contributor(s) and not of MDPI and/or the editor(s). MDPI and/or the editor(s) disclaim responsibility for any injury to people or property resulting from any ideas, methods, instructions or products referred to in the content.

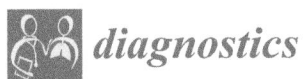

Article

Gross Cystic Disease Fluid Protein-15 (GCDFP-15) Expression Characterizes Breast Mucinous Carcinomas in Older Women

Mayumi Kinoshita [1,2], Motoji Sawabe [1,3], Yurie Soejima [1], Makiko Naka Mieno [4], Tomio Arai [5] and Naoko Honma [2,6,*]

[1] Department of Molecular Pathology, Graduate School of Medical and Dental Sciences, Tokyo Medical and Dental University, Tokyo 113-8510, Japan
[2] Department of Clinical Laboratory Medicine, Faculty of Health Science Technology, Bunkyo Gakuin University, Tokyo 113-8668, Japan
[3] Department of Diagnostic Pathology, Hitachi General Hospital, Hitachi 317-0077, Japan
[4] Department of Medical Informatics, Center for Information, Jichi Medical University, Shimotsuke 329-0498, Japan
[5] Department of Pathology, Tokyo Metropolitan Geriatric Hospital, Tokyo 173-0015, Japan
[6] Department of Pathology, Faculty of Medicine, Toho University, Tokyo 143-8540, Japan
* Correspondence: naoko.honma@med.toho-u.ac.jp

Abstract: The predominant histological subtype of breast mucinous carcinoma in older women is type B (hypercellular type), and, in younger women, it is type A (hypocellular type). The characteristics of mucinous carcinomas of the same histological subtype may differ between older and younger women. This study aims to systematically clarify the pathological/immunohistochemical features of mucinous carcinomas. A total of 21 surgical cases of mucinous carcinoma (type A/B: 9/12 cases) in the older group ($\geq$65 years) and 16 cases (type A/B: 14/2 cases) in the younger group ($\leq$55 years) (n = 37) were included. Gross cystic disease fluid protein-15 (GCDFP-15) and eight other markers were used for immunostaining. The GCDFP-15-positive rate in the older group was high regardless of the histological subtype (type A, 77.8%; type B, 91.7%). The GCDFP-15 positivity in the older group was significantly higher than that in the younger group ($p < 0.001$ for Allred score). Among type A, GCDFP-15 positivity was significantly higher in the older group than in the younger group ($p = 0.042$ for the Allred score and $p = 0.007$ for the positivity rate). The present results suggest that GCDFP-15 expression characterizes mucinous carcinomas in older women.

Keywords: breast; mucinous carcinoma; gross cystic disease fluid protein-15 (GCDFP-15); older; apocrine

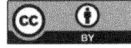

1. Introduction

Mucinous carcinoma is an invasive breast cancer histologically characterized by clusters of tumor cells suspended in extracellular mucin. Pure mucinous carcinoma is more common in older individuals and is generally associated with an excellent prognosis. Of all breast cancers, 2–4% are mucinous carcinomas, while in older women mucinous carcinomas account for more than 10% of breast cancer cases [1–4]. Histologically, pure mucinous carcinoma is classified as either type A (hypocellular: tubular, ribbon-like, and small papillary clusters with a large amount of extracellular mucin) or type B (hypercellular: large epithelial clumps or sheets with a small amount of extracellular mucin) [4,5]. Type B lesions are frequently positive for neuroendocrine markers (e.g., synaptophysin, chromogranin A, CD56) [6,7], and the surrounding tissues often have ductal carcinoma in situ (DCIS) components with a neuroendocrine tendency, which are considered precursor lesions [8].

In our previous study, approximately 16% of patients aged 85 years and older had mucinous carcinomas, and 11% had apocrine carcinomas [3]. In older patients with mucinous carcinomas, type B was predominant, as previously mentioned, and most type B lesions were positive for the apocrine marker gross cystic disease fluid protein-15 (GCDFP-15) [3,7]. Eosinophilic cytoplasm is also a characteristic cytological feature of type B lesions, which may reflect an apocrine character. Many lobular carcinomas in older patients are pleomorphic lobular carcinomas, which are referred to as apocrine-type lobular carcinomas. Type B mucinous carcinomas may also be considered apocrine-type mucinous carcinomas. For apocrine differentiated carcinomas, treatments targeting the androgen receptor (AR) have recently attracted attention due to their characteristic AR expression.

Mucinous carcinomas are generally considered hormone receptor-positive and human epidermal growth factor receptor 2 (HER2)-negative. They are the so-called luminal A-type cancers that have a favorable prognosis and a uniform clinical response [9,10]. However, genetic analysis has shown that type B mucinous carcinoma and neuroendocrine cancers have a common spectrum and a worse prognosis than type A [2]. Thus, the optimal clinical response may vary according to type A or B [11].

Type A and B mucinous carcinomas of the breast are common in younger and older women, respectively. As the hormonal environment of women varies greatly with age, even mucinous carcinomas of the same histological type may differ in their biological properties between older and younger individuals. In our previous study of mucinous carcinoma in older patients, there were special type A carcinomas with cytological features of type B carcinomas [7]. Therefore, this study aims to systematically clarify the clinicopathological features of mucinous carcinomas in older women by comparing the classical factors, such as type A/B, estrogen receptor (ER), progesterone receptor (PgR), HER2, nuclear grade, and Ki-67 score, as well as the expression of neuroendocrine and apocrine markers, with those from young to middle-aged women.

2. Materials and Methods

2.1. Subjects and Classification of Mucinous Carcinoma

The histological classification was based on the WHO classification [4]. Of the patients with surgical specimens diagnosed as pure-type mucinous carcinoma of the female breast between 2004 and 2017, 40 patients were aged 65 years and older (older group), and 16 were patients aged 55 years and younger (younger group).

Capella et al. reported that type A (hypocellular variant) has a mucus component of 60–90% while type B (hypercellular variant) has a mucus component of 33–75% [5]. In our study, to classify types A and B, specimens were evaluated by two separate pathologists. Specimen scores were obtained by scoring the cell component ratio using five levels (1: <20%, 2: 20–39%, 3: 40–59%, 4: 60–79%, 5: ≥80%), and cell cluster size was obtained by using three levels (1: small, 2: intermediate, and 3: large) and adding them [5]. Specimens with scores 2–3 and 6–8 were concordant, and they were classified as type A and type B, respectively. Cases with scores of 4 and 5 were evaluated as borderline, and when the outcome was discordant, the two pathologists reviewed the glass slides and decided together.

According to the histological type, there were 9 cases of type A and 31 cases of type B in the older group and 14 cases of type A and 2 cases of type B in the younger group (Fisher's exact test, $p < 0.001$). In the histological/immunohistochemical examination, 12 out of 31 cases of type B in the older group were available.

2.2. Clinicopathological Analysis

Pathological staging was based on UICC [12]. Nuclear grading was assessed according to the nuclear grading classification in the "Japanese Classification of Breast Cancer", which is routinely used in Japan and has been confirmed to reflect the prognosis of Japanese breast cancer patients [13,14]. Briefly, the sum of nuclear atypia (1, mild; 2, moderate; 3, severe) and mitotic counts per 10 high-power fields (1, <5; 2, 5–10; 3, >10) was classified into a nuclear grade (I, 2 or 3; II, 4; III, 5 or 6).

2.3. Immunohistochemical Procedures and Evaluations

Immunohistochemical analyses for GCDFP-15, chromogranin A (CGA), synaptophysin (SYP), CD56, AR, ER, PgR, HER2, and Ki-67 were applied to the representative slides of formalin-fixed and paraffin-embedded tissues (Table 1). After antigen retrieval (none or heat-treatment for 40 min at pH6 or pH9), the slides were incubated for 30 min with the primary antibodies GCDFP-15, CGA, SYP, CD56, AR, ER, PgR, and Ki-67. After the endogenous peroxidase was quenched with 3% H_2O_2 in distilled water, the slides were incubated with secondary antibodies and detected using Histofine Simple Stain MAX-PO (MULTI) (Nichirei Biosciences Inc., Tokyo, Japan) and DAB substrate kits (Nichirei). HER2 immunohistochemical staining was performed according to the kit's protocol (SV2-61γ, monoclonal: Nichirei).

Table 1. Experimental conditions for immunohistochemistry of breast mucinous carcinoma.

Primary Antibody	Primary Ab (Clone Name)	Dilution	Antigen Retrieval Method	Intracellular Localization	Positive Thresholds	Supplier
GCDFP-15	M (D6)	1:700	None	Cp	AS ≥ 4	SIGNET
CGA	P	RtoU	None	Cp	AS ≥ 3	Nichirei
SYP	M (27G12)	RtoU	None	Cp	AS ≥ 4	Nichirei
CD56	M (MRQ-42)	RtoU	40 min, pH 9	Cm	AS ≥ 3	Nichirei
AR	M (AR27)	1:25	40 min, pH 9	N	AS ≥ 3	Novocastra
ER	M (SPI)	RtoU	40 min, pH 9	N	AS ≥ 3	Nichirei
PgR	M (A9621A)	RtoU	40 min, pH 9	N	AS ≥ 3	Nichirei
HER2	M (SV2-61γ)	Kit	None	Cm	HS ≥ 3+	Nichirei
Ki-67	M (MIB-1)	1:200	40 min, pH 6	N	LI ≥ 5%	Dako

AR: androgen receptor; CGA: chromogranin A; ER: estrogen receptor; GCDFP-15: gross cystic disease fluid protein-15; HER2: human epidermal growth factor receptor 2; PgR: progesterone receptor; SYP: synaptophysin; Ab, antibody; M, monoclonal; P, polyclonal; RtoU, ready to use; Cp, cytoplasm; Cm, cell membrane; N, nucleus; AS, Allred score (total score); HS, HER2 score; LI, labeling index; SIGNET, SIGNET Lab, Inc., Dedham, USA; Nichirei, Nichirei Biosciences Inc., Tokyo, Japan; Novocastra, Novocastra Lab, Ltd., Sheffield UK; Dako Japan Inc., Tokyo, Japan.

To assess the staining, the percentage of immunoreactive cancerous cells was independently estimated in the nucleus (AR, ER, PgR, and Ki-67), cytoplasm (GCDFP-15, CGA, SYP, and CD56), and cytoplasmic membrane (HER2). We used the classification score proposed by Allred et al. for ER/PgR estimation in 1998 [15,16]. A positive case was defined as having an Allred score of 3 or more for CGA, CD56, AR, ER, and PgR or having a score of 4 or more for GCDFP-15 and SYP. In terms of HER2, a score of 3 was considered positive [17]. The Ki-67 score was defined as low when Ki-67-positive cells were <5% and high when Ki-67-positive cells were ≥5%. A high Ki-67 score was considered positive (Table 1).

2.4. Statistical Analyses

The Wilcoxon rank sum test was used to compare the Allred scores for each factor between the two groups. The Kruskal–Wallis test was used to compare the Allred score for each factor among the three groups. The Dunn test was used for pair-by-pair comparisons if the Kruskal–Wallis test was significant. Fisher's exact test was used for contingency tables. The level of significance was set at $p < 0.05$. SPSS Statistics version 25 (IBM, Japan, Ltd., Tokyo, Japan) was used for statistical calculations.

3. Results

3.1. Clinicopathological Features

The mean age of the patients was 81.7 ± 6.8 years (range, 67–92 years) for the older group and 44.6 ± 8.6 years (range, 28–55 years) for the younger group. The T category that accounted for 50% or more of the cases was T2 for the older group and T1 for the younger group. The older group tended to have larger tumor sizes than the younger group. There were no N2 and N3 N-stage cases, and there was no significant difference between the two groups. All patients were negative for distant metastases. The TNM stage that accounted for 50% or more of the cases was stage II for the older group and stage I for the younger group. Nuclear grading showed no significant differences (Table 2). All patients were free from recurrence.

Table 2. Clinicopathological summary of breast mucinous carcinoma.

	Older Group (≥65 y/o)	Younger Group (<55 y/o)	Fisher's Exact Test (p-Value)
Number of cases	21	16	
Age, mean ± SD	81.7 ± 6.81	44.6 ± 8.63	
(range)	(67–92)	(28–55)	
T category (%)			0.733
T0	0 (0%)	0 (0%)	
T1	7 (33.3%)	8 (50.0%)	
T2	11 (52.4%)	6 (37.5%)	
T3	3 (14.3%)	2 (12.5%)	
T4	0 (0%)	0 (0%)	
N stage			1.000
N0	18 (85.7%)	14 (87.5%)	
N1	3 (14.3%)	2 (12.5%)	
N2, N3	0 (0%)	0 (0%)	
M category			
M0	21 (100%)	16 (100%)	
M1	0 (0%)	0 (0%)	
TNM stage			0.364
Stage 0	0 (0%)	0 (0%)	
Stage I	7 (33.3%)	8 (50%)	
Stage II	13 (61.9%)	6 (37.5%)	
Stage III	1 (4.8%)	2 (12.5%)	
Stage IV	0 (0%)	0 (0%)	
Nuclear grade			0.832
Grade I	4 (19.0%)	4 (25.0%)	
Grade II	10 (47.6%)	8 (50.0%)	
Grade III	7 (33.3%)	4 (25.0%)	

SD, standard deviation.

3.2. Immunohistochemical Study

Typical histological images of each type are shown in Figure 1A,B. Typical microscopic images of GCDFP-15 immunostaining from the different age groups and carcinoma types are shown in Figure 1C–F. Additional positive immunostaining images are shown in Figure 2. The Allred scores are statistically analyzed in Tables 3–5. When the cases were divided into four groups according to age group and carcinoma type, there were only two type B cases in the younger group. Thus, the remaining three groups were compared, as shown in Tables 4 and 5.

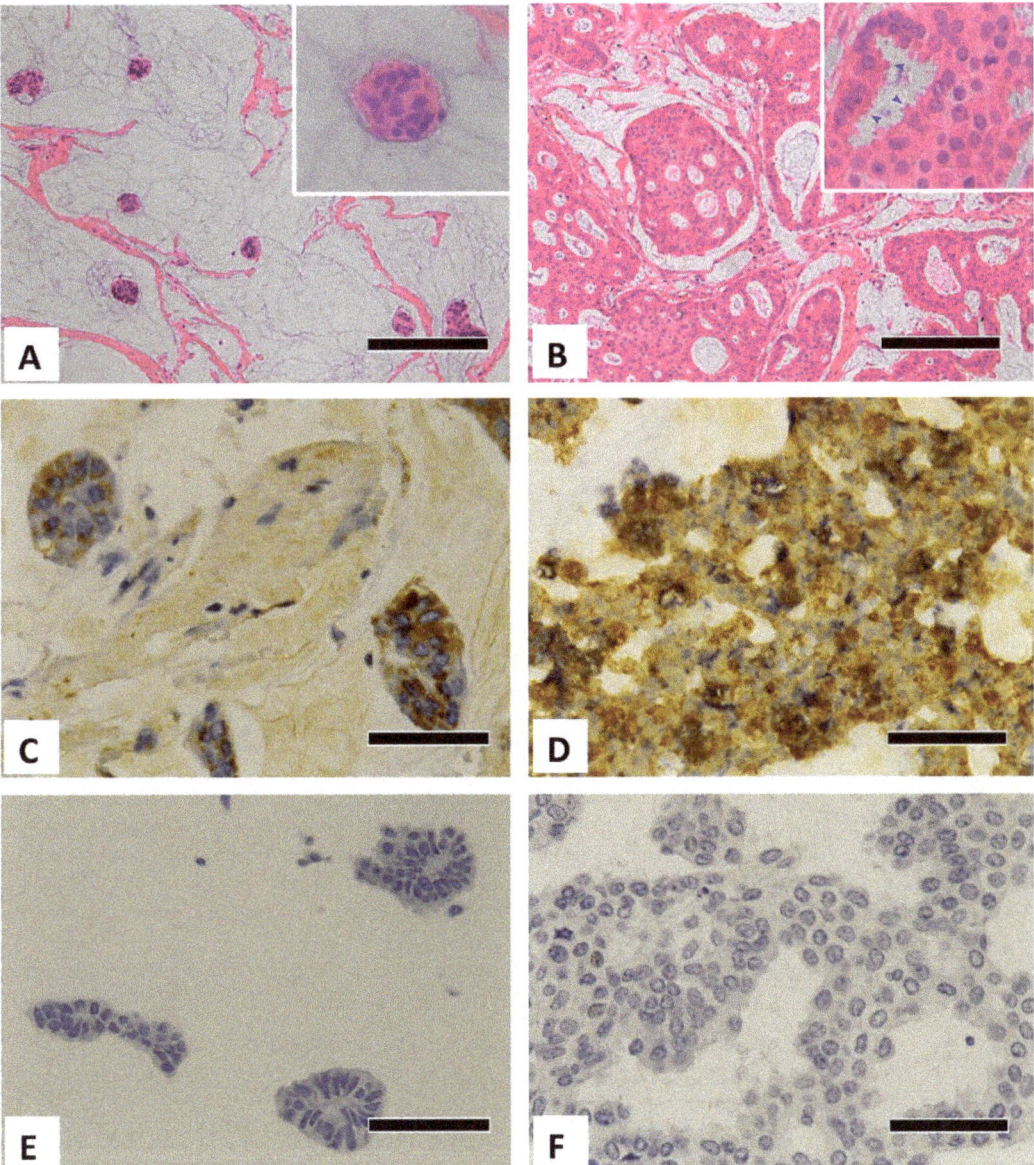

Figure 1. Microscopic pictures of breast mucinous carcinoma. (**A**) Histological image of a type A mucinous carcinoma. Note tubular and papillary small clusters with a large amount of extracellular mucin (HE stain). The inset shows a magnified image. (**B**) Histological image of a type B mucinous carcinoma. Large epithelial clumps or sheets composed of tumor cells with eosinophilic cytoplasm and a small amount of extracellular mucin (HE staining). The magnified image inset shows tumor cells with apocrine snouts (arrowheads) and abundant eosinophilic cytoplasm. (**C**) Older, type A (immunohistochemical pictures of GCDFP-15 positivity). (**D**) Older, type B (immunohistochemical pictures of GCDFP-15 positivity). (**E**) Younger, type A (immunohistochemical pictures of GCDFP-15 negativity). (**F**) Younger, type B (immunohistochemical pictures of GCDFP-15 negativity). GCDFP-15: gross cystic disease fluid protein-15. Scale bar = 200 μm (**A**,**B**), 50 μm (**C**–**F**).

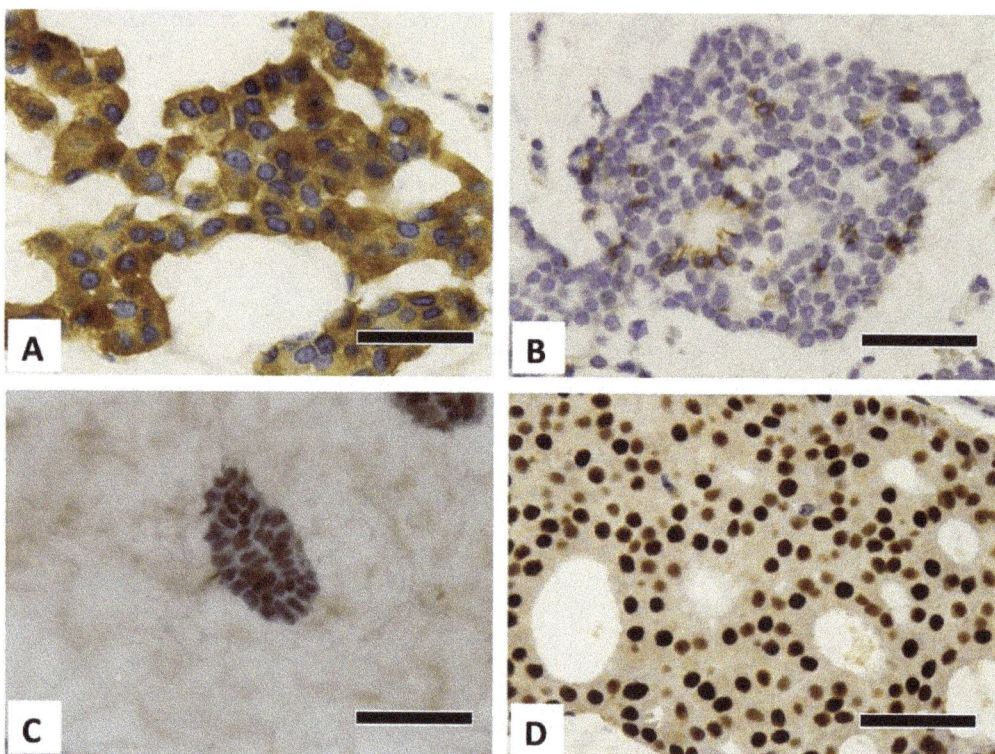

Figure 2. Immunohistochemical pictures of breast mucinous carcinoma. (**A**) SYP-positive cancer (older, type B), (**B**) CD56-positive cancer (older, type B), (**C**) AR-positive cancer (younger, type A), (**D**) AR-positive cancer (older, type B). AR, androgen receptor; SYP, synaptophysin. Scale bar = 50 μm.

Table 3. Comparisons of immunohistochemical features of breast mucinous carcinoma by age group and type.

Antibodies	Median Score (Range)			Median Score (Range)		
	Older	Younger	p-Value (Older vs. Younger)	Type A	Type B	p-Value (Type A vs. B)
Number of cases	21	16		23	14	
GCDFP-15	5 (0–8)	0 (0–5)	**<0.001**	3 (0–8)	5.5 (0–8)	**0.014**
CGA	0 (0–6)	2.5 (0–7)	**0.046**	2 (0–6)	0 (2–8)	0.394
SYP	4 (0–8)	2 (0–8)	0.059	3 (0–8)	6 (0–8)	0.186
CD56	0 (0–7)	0 (0–3)	0.201	0 (0–6)	1 (0–7)	0.237
AR	6 (3–8)	6 (2–7)	0.250	6 (4–8)	6 (2–8)	0.652
ER	8 (6–8)	7.5 (4–8)	0.906	7 (4–8)	8 (7–8)	**0.032**
PgR	6 (2–8)	7 (0–8)	0.376	6 (2–8)	5.5 (0–8)	0.525
HER2	0 (0–2)	0 (0–3)	1.000	0 (0–3)	0 (0–2)	0.904
Ki-67	1.5 (1–30)	1.5 (0–15)	0.874	1.5 (0–10)	1.75 (1–30)	0.190

p-values are calculated by the Wilcoxon rank sum test. AR: androgen receptor; CGA: chromogranin A; ER: estrogen receptor; GCDFP-15: gross cystic disease fluid protein-15; HER2: human epidermal growth receptor 2; PgR: progesterone receptor; SYP: synaptophysin.

Table 4. Immunohistochemical features of breast mucinous carcinomas among four subgroups.

Antibodies	Median Score (Range)				p-Value (1) (2) (3) (KW Test)	p-Value (1) vs. (2)/(1) vs. (3) (Dunn Test)
	Older Type A (1)	Older Type B (2)	Younger Type A (3)	Younger Type B		
Number of cases	9	12	14	2		
GCDFP-15	5 (0–8)	6 (3–8)	0 (0–5)	0, 0	**<0.001**	1.000/**0.042**
CGA	0 (0–6)	0 (0–6)	2 (0–6)	3, 7	0.124	n.a.
SYP	4 (0–8)	5 (0–8)	2 (0–5)	6, 8	**0.024**	1.000/0.093
CD56	0 (0–6)	1 (0–7)	0 (0–6)	0, 3	0.545	n.a.
AR	7 (4–8)	6 (3–8)	6 (4–7)	7, 2	0.447	n.a.
ER	7 (6–8)	8 (7–8)	7.5 (4–8)	7, 8	0.077	n.a.
PgR	6 (2–8)	5.5 (2–8)	7 (2–8)	0, 8	0.793	n.a.
HER2	0 (0–1)	0 (0–2)	0 (0–3)	0, 0	0.738	n.a.
Ki-67	1.5 (1–5)	1.5 (1–30)	1.25 (0–10)	5, 15	0.248	n.a.

p-values are calculated by the Kruskal–Wallis test and Dunn test. AR: androgen receptor; CGA: chromogranin A; ER: estrogen receptor; GCDFP-15: gross cystic disease fluid protein-15; HER2: human epidermal growth receptor 2; KW test: Kruskal–Wallis test; PgR: progesterone receptor; SYP: synaptophysin; n.a.: not applicable.

Table 5. Immunohistochemical features of carcinomas among four subgroups.

Antibodies	Older Type A (1)	Older Type B (2)	Younger Type A (3)	Younger Type B	p-Value (1) vs. (2)/(1) vs. (3)
	n = 9 +/−	n = 12 +/−	n = 14 +/−	n = 2 +/−	
GCDFP-15	7/2	11/1	2/12	0/2	0.553/**0.007**
CGA	4/5	3/9	6/8	2/0	0.397/1.000
SYP	6/3	7/5	3/11	2/0	1.000/0.077
CD56	3/6	5/7	2/12	1/1	1.000/0.343
AR	8/0	10/0	14/0	1/1	1.000/1.000
ER	9/0	12/0	14/0	2/0	1.000/1.000
PgR	8/1	10/2	12/2	1/1	1.000/1.000
HER2	0/9	0/12	1/13	0/2	1.000/1.000
Ki-67	1/8	3/9	4/10	2/0	0.603/0.611

p-values were calculated using Fisher's exact test. AR: androgen receptor; CGA: chromogranin A; ER: estrogen receptor; GCDFP-15: gross cystic disease fluid protein-15; HER2: human epidermal growth receptor 2; PgR: progesterone receptor; SYP: synaptophysin.

3.2.1. GCDFP-15

The Allred scores were significantly higher in the older group than in the younger group ($p < 0.001$), and they were significantly higher in type B carcinoma than in type A ($p = 0.014$) (Table 3). They were also significantly different among the three groups ($p < 0.001$), as shown in Table 4. No significant difference was observed between the older type A and older type B groups ($p = 1.000$), whereas a significant difference was observed between the older type A and younger type A groups ($p = 0.042$). In the dichotomous positive/negative comparison, GCDFP-15-positive expression was seen in 18 of 21 cases in the older group (85.7%) and 2 of 16 in the younger group (12.5%), yielding significant differences ($p < 0.001$). In the older group, 7 of 9 type A cases (77.8%) and 11 of 12 type B cases (91.7%) were positive for GCDFP-15, indicating a high positivity rate regardless of the carcinoma type ($p = 0.553$, Table 5. Figure 1C–F). Among type A, the positivity rate was significantly higher in the older group than in the younger group ($p = 0.007$).

3.2.2. Neuroendocrine Markers

The Allred score for CGA was lower in the older group than in the younger group ($p = 0.046$) (Table 3), however, other CGA tests showed no significant differences (Tables 4 and 5).

The Allred scores for SYP were insignificantly higher in the older group than in the younger group ($p = 0.059$) (Table 3). The difference was significant among the three groups ($p = 0.024$) (Table 4), however, no significant difference was obtained by pair-by-pair comparisons. The dichotomous analyses for SYP did not yield significant differences (Table 5).

CD56 did not differ significantly in any comparison (Tables 3–5).

3.2.3. Steroid Hormone Receptors

There were no significant differences in the AR Allred scores between the older and younger patients ($p = 0.250$) or between type A and type B ($p = 0.652$) (Table 3) and in any further analyses (Tables 4 and 5).

The ER Allred scores did not significantly differ between older and younger patients ($p = 0.906$) but were significantly higher in type B carcinoma than in type A ($p = 0.032$) (Table 3). No significant differences were found in further studies (Tables 4 and 5). The PgR Allred scores did not differ significantly in any studies (Tables 3–5).

3.2.4. HER2 and Ki-67 Immunostaining

There were no significant differences in the expression of HER2 and Ki-67 in any comparison (Tables 3–5).

3.2.5. Comparison between GCDFP-15 Expression and Other Factors

Figure 3 shows the relationships between GCDFP-15 expression and the type of mucinous carcinoma or the expression of other immunohistochemical markers considering age. Most of the mucinous carcinomas in older patients were GCDFP-15-positive irrespective of other factors, whereas those in younger patients exhibited opposite results.

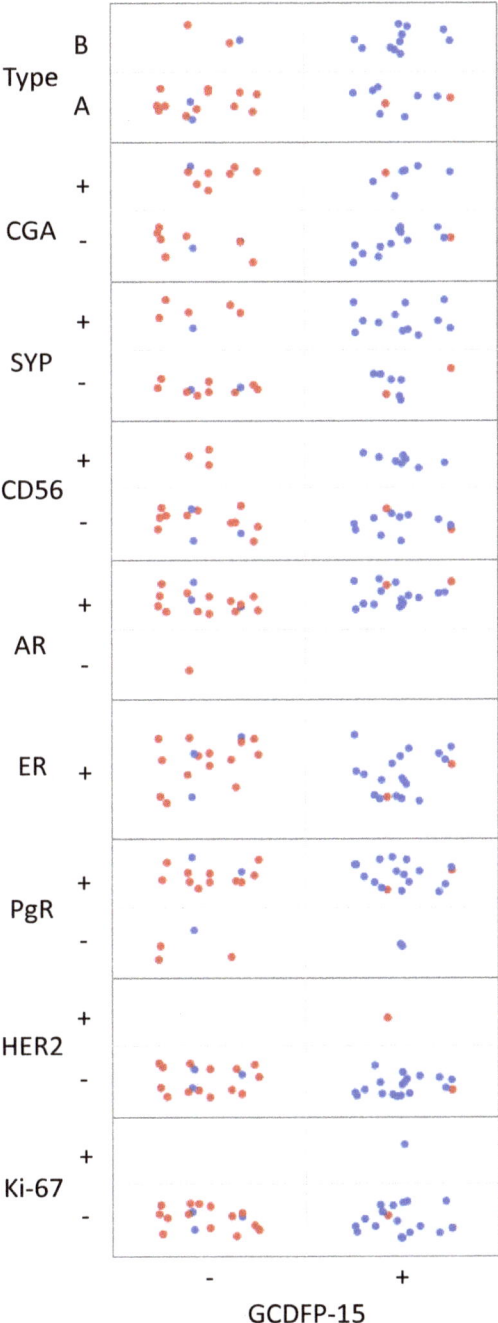

Figure 3. The relationships between GCDFP-15 expression and type of mucinous carcinoma or the expression of other immunohistochemical markers considering age (older patients in blue and younger patients in red). AR: androgen receptor; CGA: chromogranin A; ER: estrogen receptor; GCDFP-15: gross cystic disease fluid protein-15; HER2: human epidermal growth receptor 2; PgR: progesterone receptor; SYP: synaptophysin.

4. Discussion

Our results showed that GCDFP-15 expression clearly characterizes mucinous carcinoma in older patients regardless of the mucinous carcinoma subtype or the other immunohistochemical markers. The neuroendocrine character was not necessarily characteristic of mucinous carcinoma of type B or in older patients.

4.1. Apocrine Markers (GCDFP-15/AR)

We previously reported, in older patients, a high rate of mucinous and apocrine cancers and higher rates of GCDFP-15 and AR-positive cancers [3]. In the present study, mucinous carcinomas in older patients were mostly positive for both GCDFP-15 and AR and showed abundant eosinophilic cytoplasm or apocrine snouts, suggesting their apocrine-like characteristics (Figure 1). Although apocrine metaplasia in mucinous carcinomas is described in the WHO classification [18], we clearly showed for the first time that GCDFP-15 positivity was more prevalent in older patients. So far, mucinous carcinoma in older patients has been characterized by type B morphology or neuroendocrine features; however, our results demonstrated that GCDFP-15 expression most clearly characterizes the mucinous carcinoma of older patients. Pleomorphic invasive lobular carcinoma, often GCDFP-15/AR-positive and regarded as an apocrine-type invasive lobular carcinoma, is frequent in older women [18–21]. As for tumors in the other organs, about 5% of lung adenocarcinoma were reported to be positive for GCDFP-15, and most of them occurred in older individuals [22,23]. Of note, GCDFP-15 has been reportedly positive for a mucin-rich variant of salivary duct carcinoma [24] and endocrine mucin-producing sweat gland carcinoma [25], both of which commonly affects older patients, suggesting a similar phenomenon in the other organs.

Interestingly, the type A mucinous carcinomas of older individuals also exhibited apocrine-like immunohistochemical characteristics (GCDFP-15 positivity and AR positivity). The relationship between type B carcinomas and neuroendocrine characteristics is well known. However, the apocrine-like characteristic was not limited to type B carcinomas, as de Andrade Natal reported [6] but rather was found in either type of mucinous carcinoma in older patients. Conversely, type A carcinomas in older patients might differ in their biological characteristics from type A carcinomas in younger patients. We conclude that the biologically essential features of mucinous carcinomas in older patients are apocrine-like immunohistochemical features (GCDFP-15/AR positivity), rather than neuroendocrine features. Of note, apocrine differentiation is generally characterized by GCDFP-15 positivity, AR positivity, ER negativity, and PgR negativity [18]. Almost all intraductal and invasive apocrine carcinomas are positive for GCDFP-15/AR and negative for ER and PgR [26]. Most mucinous carcinomas are ER-positive and PgR-positive, regardless of patient age and histological type, and thus they are not entirely apocrine-differentiated carcinomas—they partially have apocrine character. Interestingly, GCDFP-15 tended to be negative in younger patients despite AR positivity. These points are discussed further below.

4.2. GCDFP-15 and AR/PgR Expression

The expression of GCDFP-15 is induced by AR activation caused by the binding of androgens, such as testosterone or dihydrotestosterone, to AR [27]. In our study, there was no significant difference in the expression of AR between older and younger patients. Frequent expression of AR in mucinous carcinomas was previously reported; de Andrade Natal et al. reported that AR positivity was seen in 5 of 16 cases (31.6%) of type A breast mucinous carcinomas and 13 of 23 cases (56.5%) of type B breast mucinous carcinomas [6]. Cho et al. reported that the rate of AR positivity was 21.7% in breast mucinous carcinomas, of which 47.8% of all patients were 50 years old or older [28]. AR positivity is generally higher in luminal cancers (ER/PgR-positive cancers), and it may be reasonable that mucinous cancers with higher ER/PgR positivity have higher AR positivity. However, it is worth noting that, unlike in older patients, GCDFP-15 positivity was low in younger patients despite high AR positivity. As AR is structurally similar to PgR, progesterone has the ability to bind AR and inhibits its action [29,30]. AR action may be inhibited in younger patients due to their higher blood progesterone levels. The reduced GCDFP-15 expression in younger women might be a result of progesterone binding to the AR. Blood androgen levels decrease with age, albeit at a slow rate, whereas progesterone levels decrease sharply after menopause [31–34]. In older individuals, the androgen/progesterone ratio is higher than that in younger individuals. AR is less inhibited in the older groups, and this may maintain the GCDFP-15 expression. Consequently, GCDFP-15 positivity may have been higher in older patients than in younger patients. GCDFP-15 can be an indicator of normal androgen-AR signaling, as PgR is for ER; then, it may be revealed to work as a predictor of AR-targeting therapy in the future.

4.3. Expression of Other Immunohistochemical Markers

Previous reports showed a neuroendocrine feature in type B mucinous carcinomas [6,7,35]. Our results showed that SYP positivity in older women tended to be higher than that in younger individuals (Table 3), and that it was different among three groups ($p = 0.024$) (Table 4). In contrast, the CGA positivity was significantly higher in younger women than in older women and was not significantly different between type A and type B (Table 3) or in any other comparisons (Tables 4 and 5). CD56 did not significantly differ in any comparison. Both SYP and CGA are good neuroendocrine markers with high sensitivity and specificity; however, the results of these neuroendocrine markers were inconsistent. Neuroendocrine features can also be examined by an electron microscope. Previous studies on mucinous carcinoma showed controversial results regarding the presence of neuroendocrine granules, suggesting "pseudo" neuroendocrine differentiation [36,37]. Thus, further studies are warranted to elucidate this neuroendocrine marker discrepancy.

Our immunohistochemical findings for ER, PgR, HER2, and Ki-67 suggested mucinous carcinomas were nearly all luminal A. A summary of previous reports is presented in Table 6. In all studies, more than 90% were positive for ER, and more than 80% were positive for PgR in most studies. The HER2 positivity rate was also low [1,6,38,39]. Our results were almost consistent with those reports regarding ER, PgR, and HER2. It is difficult to compare the results of Ki-67 as the Ki-67 index threshold is not universally standardized.

Table 6. Reported immunohistochemical property of breast mucinous carcinoma.

Study	Group	Number of Cases	Mean Age	ER	PgR	HER2	Ki-67	Ki-67 Threshold
Our study	Older (67–92 y/o)	21	81.7	100%	85.7%	0%	19%	5%
	Younger (28–55 y/o)	16	44.6	100%	81.3%	6.3%	37.5%	5%
Li et al. [1]	50–89 y/o	2730	n.a.	96%	83%	n.a.	n.a.	n.a.
	30–49 y/o	516	n.a.	91%	81%	n.a.	n.a.	n.a.
Di Saverio et al. [38]	25–85 y/o	11422	68.3	94.1%	81.5%	n.a.	n.a.	n.a.
de Andrade Natal et al. [6]	Type A	17	57.0	100%	52.9%	5.9%	0%	14%
	Type B	23	66.0	95.7%	73.9%	4.3%	21.7%	14%
Lacroix-Triki et al. [39]		35	n.a.	100%	85.7%	2.9%	8.6%	10%

ER, estrogen receptor; HER2, human epidermal growth receptor 2; PgR, progesterone receptor; n.a., not available.

4.4. Limitations of This Study

The small sample size of our study necessitates studies with larger sample sizes to validate our results.

5. Conclusions

Our results showed that mucinous carcinomas in older patients are more clearly characterized by GCDFP-15 expression than type B or neuroendocrine differentiation, which has been considered to characterize them.

Author Contributions: Conceptualization, N.H.; methodology, M.K., M.S. and N.H.; validation, M.K., M.N.M. and M.S.; investigation, M.K., T.A. and N.H.; resources, T.A.; data curation, M.K.; writing—original draft preparation, M.K., M.S. and N.H.; writing—review and editing, Y.S., M.S. and N.H.; visualization, M.K., M.S. and N.H.; supervision, M.S. and N.H.; project administration, M.S. and N.H.; funding acquisition, N.H. All authors have read and agreed to the published version of the manuscript.

Funding: This research was funded by JSPS/MEXT KAKENHI grant number 16K08660.

Institutional Review Board Statement: This study was conducted in accordance with the Declaration of Helsinki and approved by the Tokyo Metropolitan Geriatric Hospital Institutional Research Board (R16-19, 26 August 2016) and the Toho University Faculty of Medicine Ethics Committee (A19061_A16078_27132, 13 December 2019).

Informed Consent Statement: Informed opt-out consent was obtained from all subjects involved in this study.

Data Availability Statement: No applicable.

Acknowledgments: The authors are grateful to Tetuo Mikami, Kayo Tsuburaya, and Maho Yokoyama from the Department of Pathology, Kazutoshi Shibuya, and the staff of the Department of Surgical Pathology, Toho University Faculty of Medicine, for their valuable assistance. We also thank the staff of the Department of Pathology, Tokyo Metropolitan Geriatric Hospital, for supporting this study.

Conflicts of Interest: The authors declare no conflict of interest.

References

1. Li, C.I.; Uribe, D.J.; Daling, J.R. Clinical Characteristics of Different Histologic Types of Breast Cancer. *Br. J. Cancer* **2005**, *93*, 1046–1052. [CrossRef]
2. Komaki, K.; Sakamoto, G.; Sugano, H.; Morimoto, T.; Monden, Y. Mucinous Carcinoma of the Breast in Japan. A Prognostic Analysis Based on Morphologic Features. *Cancer* **1988**, *61*, 989–996. [CrossRef] [PubMed]
3. Honma, N.; Sakamoto, G.; Akiyama, F.; Esaki, Y.; Sawabe, M.; Arai, T.; Hosoi, T.; Harada, N.; Younes, M.; Takubo, K. Breast Carcinoma in Women Over the Age of 85: Distinct Histological Pattern and Androgen, Oestrogen, and Progesterone Receptor Status. *Histopathology* **2003**, *42*, 120–127. [CrossRef] [PubMed]
4. Wen, H.Y.; Desmedt, C.; Reis-Filho, J.S.; Schmitt, F. Mucinous carcinoma. In *Breast Tumours (WHO Classification of Tumours)*, 5th ed.; International Agency for Research on Cancer: Lyon, France, 2019; pp. 123–125.
5. Capella, C.; Eusebi, V.; Mann, B.; Azzopardi, J.G. Endocrine Differentiation in Mucoid Carcinoma of the Breast. *Histopathology* **1980**, *4*, 613–630. [CrossRef] [PubMed]
6. de Andrade Natal, R.; Derchain, S.F.; Pavanello, M.; Paiva, G.R.; Sarian, L.O.; Vassallo, J. Expression of Unusual Immunohistochemical Markers in Mucinous Breast Carcinoma. *Acta Histochem.* **2017**, *119*, 327–336. [CrossRef]
7. Shirahata, H.; Honma, N.; Kotani, T.; Imaizumi, M.; Hamashima, Y.; Esaki, Y.; Kinoshita, M.; Suzuki, A.; Sakurai, U.; Arai, T. Cytological Characteristics of Mucinous Carcinoma of the Breast in the Elderly with Bibliographical Considerations (in Japanese with English Abstract). *J. Jpn. Soc. Clin. Cytol.* **2017**, *56*, 75–84. [CrossRef]
8. Kryvenko, O.N.; Chitale, D.A.; Yoon, J.; Arias-Stella, J.; Meier, F.A.; Lee, M.W. Precursor Lesions of Mucinous Carcinoma of the Breast: Analysis of 130 Cases. *Am. J. Surg. Pathol.* **2013**, *37*, 1076–1084. [CrossRef]
9. Corben, A.D.; Brogi, E. Mucinous carcinoma. In *Rosen's Breast Pathology*, 4th ed.; Hoda, S.A., Brogi, E., Koemer, F.C., Rosen, P.P., Eds.; Lippincott Willams & Wilkins: Philadelphia, PA, USA, 2014; pp. 611–644.
10. Budzik, M.P.; Fudalej, M.M.; Badowska-Kozakiewicz, A.M. Histopathological Analysis of Mucinous Breast Cancer Subtypes and Comparison with Invasive Carcinoma of no Special Type. *Sci. Rep.* **2021**, *11*, 5770. [CrossRef]
11. Weigelt, B.; Geyer, F.C.; Horlings, H.M.; Kreike, B.; Halfwerk, H.; Reis-Filho, J.S. Mucinous and Neuroendocrine Breast Carcinomas are Transcriptionally Distinct from Invasive Ductal Carcinomas of no Special Type. *Mod. Pathol.* **2009**, *22*, 1401–1414. [CrossRef]
12. Brierley, J.D.; Gospodarowicz, M.K.; Wittekind, C. Breast Tumours. In *TNM Classification of Malignant Tumours*, 8th ed.; Brierley, J.D., Gospodarowicz, M.K., Wittekind, C., Eds.; Wiley-Blackwell: Hoboken, NJ, USA, 2017; pp. 151–158.
13. Tsuda, H.; Akiyama, F.; Kurosumi, M.; Sakamoto, G.; Watanabe, T. Establishment of Histological Criteria for High-Risk Node-Negative Breast Carcinoma for a Multi-Institutional Randomized Clinical Trial of Adjuvant Therapy. Japan National Surgical Adjuvant Study of Breast Cancer (NSAS-BC) Pathology Section. *Jpn. J. Clin. Oncol.* **1998**, *28*, 486–491. [CrossRef]
14. Otsuki, Y.; Shimizu, S.; Suwa, K.; Yoshida, M.; Kanzaki, M.; Kobayashi, H. Which is the Better Pathological Prognostic Factor, the Nottingham Histological Grade Or the Japanese Nuclear Grade? A Large Scale Study with a Long-Term Follow-Up. *Jpn. J. Clin. Oncol.* **2007**, *37*, 266–274. [CrossRef] [PubMed]
15. Fitzgibbons, P.L.; Dillon, D.A.; Alsabeh, R.; Berman, M.A.; Hayes, D.F.; Hicks, D.G.; Hughes, K.S.; Nofech-Mozes, S. Template for Reporting Results of Biomarker Testing of Specimens from Patients with Carcinoma of the Breast. *Arch. Pathol. Lab. Med.* **2014**, *138*, 595–601. [CrossRef] [PubMed]

16. Soares, M.; Madeira, S.; Correia, J.; Peleteiro, M.; Cardoso, F.; Ferreira, F. Molecular Based Subtyping of Feline Mammary Carcinomas and Clinicopathological Characterization. *Breast* **2016**, *27*, 44–51. [CrossRef]
17. Tsuda, H.; Akiyama, F.; Terasaki, H.; Hasegawa, T.; Kurosumi, M.; Shimadzu, M.; Yamamori, S.; Sakamoto, G. Detection of HER-2/Neu (C-Erb B-2) DNA Amplification in Primary Breast Carcinoma. Interobserver Reproducibility and Correlation with Immunohistochemical HER-2 Overexpression. *Cancer* **2001**, *92*, 2965–2974. [CrossRef] [PubMed]
18. Provenzano, E.; Gatalica, Z.; Vranic, S. Carcinoma with apocrine differentiation. In *Breast Tumours (WHO Classification of Tumours)*, 5th ed.; International Agency for Research on Cancer: Lyon, France, 2019; pp. 131–133.
19. Kasashima, S.; Kawashima, A.; Zen, Y.; Ozaki, S.; Kobayashi, M.; Tsujibata, A.; Minato, H. Expression of Aberrant Mucins in Lobular Carcinoma with Histiocytoid Feature of the Breast. *Virchows Arch.* **2007**, *450*, 397–403. [CrossRef]
20. Shimizu, S.; Kitamura, H.; Ito, T.; Nakamura, T.; Fujisawa, J.; Matsukawa, H. Histiocytoid Breast Carcinoma: Histological, Immunohistochemical, Ultrastructural, Cytological and Clinicopathological Studies. *Pathol. Int.* **1998**, *48*, 549–556. [CrossRef]
21. Tan, P.H.; Harada, O.; Thike, A.A.; Tse, G.M. Histiocytoid Breast Carcinoma: An Enigmatic Lobular Entity. *J. Clin. Pathol.* **2011**, *64*, 654–659. [CrossRef]
22. Striebel, J.M.; Dacic, S.; Yousem, S.A. Gross Cystic Disease Fluid Protein-(GCDFP-15): Expression in Primary Lung Adenocarcinoma. *Am. J. Surg. Pathol.* **2008**, *32*, 426–432. [CrossRef] [PubMed]
23. Wang, L.J.; Greaves, W.O.; Sabo, E.; Noble, L.; Tavares, R.; Ng, T.; DeLellis, R.A.; Resnick, M.B. GCDFP-15 Positive and TTF-1 Negative Primary Lung Neoplasms: A Tissue Microarray Study of 381 Primary Lung Tumors. *Appl. Immunohistochem. Mol. Morphol.* **2009**, *17*, 505–511. [CrossRef]
24. Simpson, R.H.W.; Prasad, A.R.; Lewis, J.E.; Skálová, A.; David, L. Mucin-Rich Variant of Salivary Duct Carcinoma: A Clinicopathologic and Immunohistochemical Study of Four Cases. *Am. J. Surg. Pathol.* **2003**, *27*, 1070–1079. [CrossRef]
25. Ravi, P.Y.; Walsh, N.M.; Archibald, C.; Pasternak, S. Endocrine Mucin-Producing Sweat Gland Carcinoma: Emerging Evidence of Multicentric Cutaneous Origin and Occasional Concurrence with Analogous Breast Tumors. *Am. J. Dermatopathol.* **2022**, *44*, 321–326. [CrossRef] [PubMed]
26. Brogi, E. Apocrine carcinoma. In *Rosen's Breast Pathology*, 4th ed.; Hoda, S., Brogi, E., Koerner, F.C., Rosen, P.P., Eds.; Wolters Kluwer Health, Inc.: Philadelphia, PA, USA, 2014; pp. 645–666.
27. Loos, S.; Schulz, K.D.; Hackenberg, R. Regulation of GCDFP-15 Expression in Human Mammary Cancer Cells. *Int. J. Mol. Med.* **1999**, *4*, 135–140. [CrossRef]
28. Cho, L.; Hsu, Y. Expression of Androgen, Estrogen and Progesterone Receptors in Mucinous Carcinoma of the Breast. *Kaohsiung J. Med. Sci.* **2008**, *24*, 227–232. [CrossRef]
29. Raudrant, D.; Rabe, T. Progestogens with Antiandrogenic Properties. *Drugs* **2003**, *63*, 463–492. [CrossRef] [PubMed]
30. Bardin, C.W.; Brown, T.; Isomaa, V.V.; Jänne, O.A. Progestins can Mimic, Inhibit and Potentiate the Actions of Androgens. *Pharmacol. Ther.* **1983**, *23*, 443–459. [CrossRef]
31. Hankinson, S.E.; Eliassen, A.H. Endogenous Estrogen, Testosterone and Progesterone Levels in Relation to Breast Cancer Risk. *J. Steroid Biochem. Mol. Biol.* **2007**, *106*, 24–30. [CrossRef] [PubMed]
32. Manjer, J.; Johansson, R.; Berglund, G.; Janzon, L.; Kaaks, R.; Agren, A.; Lenner, P. Postmenopausal Breast Cancer Risk in Relation to Sex Steroid Hormones, Prolactin and SHBG (Sweden). *Cancer Causes Control* **2003**, *14*, 599–607. [CrossRef] [PubMed]
33. Missmer, S.A.; Eliassen, A.H.; Barbieri, R.L.; Hankinson, S.E. Endogenous Estrogen, Androgen, and Progesterone Concentrations and Breast Cancer Risk among Postmenopausal Women. *J. Natl. Cancer Inst.* **2004**, *96*, 1856–1865. [CrossRef]
34. Sieri, S.; Krogh, V.; Bolelli, G.; Abagnato, C.A.; Grioni, S.; Pala, V.; Evangelista, A.; Allemani, C.; Micheli, A.; Tagliabue, G.; et al. Sex Hormone Levels, Breast Cancer Risk, and Cancer Receptor Status in Postmenopausal Women: The ORDET Cohort. *Cancer Epidemiol. Biomark. Prev.* **2009**, *18*, 169–176. [CrossRef]
35. Scopsi, L.; Andreola, S.; Pilotti, S.; Bufalino, R.; Baldini, M.T.; Testori, A.; Rilke, F. Mucinous Carcinoma of the Breast. A Clinicopathologic, Histochemical, and Immunocytochemical Study with Special Reference to Neuroendocrine Differentiation. *Am. J. Surg. Pathol.* **1994**, *18*, 702–711. [CrossRef]
36. Dickersin, G.R.; Maluf, H.M.; Koerner, F.C. Solid Papillary Carcinoma of Breast: An Ultrastructural Study. *Ultrastruct. Pathol.* **1997**, *21*, 153–161. [CrossRef] [PubMed]
37. Ng, W. Mammary Mucinous Carcinoma with Marked Cytoplasmic Hyalinization. A Report of 2 Cases with Emphasis on Fine Needle Aspiration Cytologic Findings. *Acta Cytol.* **2003**, *47*, 1045–1049. [CrossRef] [PubMed]
38. Di Saverio, S.; Gutierrez, J.; Avisar, E. A Retrospective Review with Long Term Follow Up of 11.400 Cases of Pure Mucinous Breast Carcinoma. *Breast Cancer Res. Treat.* **2008**, *111*, 541–547. [CrossRef] [PubMed]
39. Lacroix-Triki, M.; Suarez, P.H.; MacKay, A.; Lambros, M.B.; Natrajan, R.; Savage, K.; Geyer, F.C.; Weigelt, B.; Ashworth, A.; Reis-Filho, J.S. Mucinous Carcinoma of the Breast is Genomically Distinct from Invasive Ductal Carcinomas of no Special Type. *J. Pathol.* **2010**, *222*, 282–298. [CrossRef]

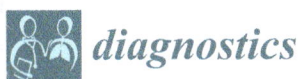

Review

The Female Reproductive Tract Microbiome and Cancerogenesis: A Review Story of Bacteria, Hormones, and Disease

Oana Gabriela Trifanescu [1,2,†], Raluca Alexandra Trifanescu [3,4,†], Radu Iulian Mitrica [1,2,*], Diana Maria Bran [2,†], Georgia Luiza Serbanescu [1,2,*], Laurentiu Valcauan [2], Serban Andrei Marinescu [5,†], Laurentia Nicoleta Gales [1,6], Bogdan Cosmin Tanase [7] and Rodica Maricela Anghel [1,2]

1. Department of Oncology, „Carol Davila" University of Medicine and Pharmacy, 022328 Bucharest, Romania
2. 2nd Department of Radiotherapy, „Prof. Dr. Al. Trestioreanu" Institute of Oncology; 022328 Bucharest, Romania
3. Department of Endocrinology, "Carol Davila" University of Medicine and Pharmacy, 011863 Bucharest, Romania
4. "C.I. Parhon" Institute of Endocrinology, 011863 Bucharest, Romania
5. Department of Surgery, „Prof. Dr. Al. Trestioreanu" Institute of Oncology, 022328 Bucharest, Romania
6. 2nd Department of Oncology, „Prof. Dr. Al. Trestioreanu" Institute of Oncology, 022328 Bucharest, Romania
7. Department of Thoracic Surgery, "Prof. Dr. Al. Trestioreanu" Institute of Oncology, 022328 Bucharest, Romania
* Correspondence: radu.mitrica@umfcd.ro (R.I.M.); luiza.serbanescu@umfcd.ro (G.L.S.)
† These authors contributed equally to this work.

Abstract: The microbiota is the complex community of microorganisms that populate a particular environment in the human body, whereas the microbiome is defined by the entire habitat—microorganisms and their environment. The most abundant and, therefore, the most studied microbiome is that of the gastrointestinal tract. However, the microbiome of the female reproductive tract is an interesting research avenue, and this article explores its role in disease development. The vagina is the reproductive organ that hosts the largest number of bacteria, with a healthy profile represented mainly by *Lactobacillus* spp. On the other hand, the female upper reproductive tract (uterus, Fallopian tubes, ovaries) contains only a very small number of bacteria. Previously considered sterile, recent studies have shown the presence of a small microbiota here, but there are still debates on whether this is a physiologic or pathologic occurrence. Of particular note is that estrogen levels significantly influence the composition of the microbiota of the female reproductive tract. More and more studies show a link between the microbiome of the female reproductive tract and the development of gynecological cancers. This article reviews some of these findings.

Keywords: microbiome; carcinogenesis; female reproductive tract; immunotherapy

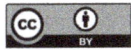

1. Introduction

1.1. The Microbiome of the Female Reproductive Tract

The healthy vagina harbors a microbiota characterized by a low diversity of species, represented mainly by *Lactobacillus* spp. (*Lactobacillus crispatus, Lactobacillus gasseri, Lactobacillus iners, Lactobacillus jensenii, Lactobacillus vaginalis*) [1–3]. This starkly contrasts with the high diversity of species demonstrated by the healthy colon [3–6]. The vagina contains species that process glycogen and its breakdown products to produce lactic acid, thus leading to an acidic pH of less than 4.5 [7]. This is important because it inactivates pathogens and prevents the ascent of pathogenic bacteria to the upper reproductive tract. Lactobacilli also secrete antimicrobial products and prevent the adhesion of pathogens [8].

On the pathological side, endometriosis, gynecological cancers and fertility problems may all be related to uterine microbiota [3].

Vaginal dysbiosis is characterized by a high diversity of bacterial species and a high pH. A diseased vaginal environment contains a mixture of anaerobic bacteria such as

Sneathia spp., *Atopobium* spp., *Porphyromonas* spp., *Gardnerella vaginalis* etc. It can sometimes contain bacteria such as *Streptococcus* spp., *Staphylococcus* spp. and *Enterobacteriaceae*. In vaginal dysbiosis, the *Lactobacillus* spp. are low in number leading to an increased risk of bacterial vaginosis. The specific types of lactobacilli also matter. For instance, a vagina that contains mainly *Lactobacillus iners* frequently transitions to become anaerobe-dominant [2,9]. However, not all *Lactobacillus* species have the same effect; for example, this transition fails to develop in a vagina with predominant *Lactobacillus crispatus*. This might be related to the type of lactic acid produced by each bacterium. *Lactobacillus iners* only synthesizes the L-isoform of lactic acid, which correlates with higher levels of metalloproteinases in vaginal secretions and lesser epithelial integrity of the vaginal wall [2,10]. This is of practical importance in deciding the appropriate *Lactobacillus* spp. to use as vaginal probiotics.

The upper female reproductive tract (uterus, Fallopian tubes and ovaries) was considered sterile for a long time. Recent molecular studies showed that it might harbor its own microbiota, but it is unclear if the samples used in studies were not contaminated during collection [2]. The healthy upper reproductive tract would contain only a very small biomass of bacteria whose composition and implication for the woman's and baby's health is under investigation. This biomass's exact composition and diversity are still scrutinized, but it would probably contain a smaller percentage of lactobacilli than the vagina.

In contrast, the diseased and pathologic upper reproductive tract often contains a large biomass. Among the bacteria that colonize the upper genital tract, some can be particularly aggressive, leading to infertility, such as *Chlamydia*, *Mycoplasma*, *Acinetobacter*, and *Brucella*. On the other hand, certain bacteria, such as *Atopobium* and *Porphyromonas*, have been shown to correlate with endometrial hyperplasia and endometrial cancer [2]. These bacteria usually colonize the upper reproductive tract by ascending from the vagina, but there may also be direct hematogenous seeding [3].

In addition to the female reproductive tract there are two other important female microbiomes, and they all influence each other. The other two microbiomes are that of the urethra and bladder, and that of the anus and rectum. The composition of each organ's microbiota is influenced by the direct transfer of microorganisms from the other organs. Both the urethra and rectum contain *Lactobacillus* spp. [11].

1.2. Estrogens and the Estrobolome

In addition to the reproductive tract flora, another major component that influences the reproductive tract environment is represented by the female hormones, particularly estrogens. This part of the article explores the link between estrogens and the microbiome.

Estrogens are conjugated in the liver by sulfotransferase and uridine diphosphate—glucuronosyltransferase enzymes and then excreted into the gut through the bile. In the gut, some conjugated estrogens are deconjugated by beta-glucuronidase and beta-glucosidase and then reabsorbed through the intestinal epithelium back into the bloodstream [2]. Interestingly, these enzymes can be produced by some gut bacteria. Thus, the gut microbiota's composition directly impacts circulating estrogen levels [12,13].

The estrobolome is nowadays defined as the aggregate of all enteric bacterial genes whose products are capable of metabolizing estrogens [2].

The activity of different enzymes, such as β-glucuronidase, is encoded mainly by two genes. First is Gus, found in Firmicutes [14], and second is BG, found in Bacteroidetes [15]. β-glucuronidase activity is also influenced by diet [16]. A high-fat diet may increase bile acid secretion, promoting Proteobacteria growth and reducing Bacteroidetes and Firmicutes [17].

Increases in β-glucuronidase-producing Proteobacteria increase intestinal deconjugation of estrogens and estrogens levels in circulation. This mechanism is intensified in obese patients, mainly due to peripheral aromatization of testosterone and androstenedione to estradiol and estrone [18,19].

Since estrogen levels are associated with various types of cancers, such as endometrial or breast cancer, we can hypothesize that the estrobolome also impacts the carcinogenesis of these types of cancers.

Moreover, the composition of the vaginal microbiome is deeply impacted by estrogen levels. Before puberty and after menopause, the vaginal microbiome consists primarily of anaerobes, whereas for healthy females of reproductive age, the vaginal microbiome consists mainly of *Lactobacillus* spp. [8,20]. Indeed, estrogens stimulate the production and secretion of glycogen by the vaginal epithelium, promoting the growth of lactobacilli. Lactobacilli then use glycogen as a food source and degrade it through fermentation. Large amounts of the lactic acid result as a final product of this process [2,8,21].

Therefore, we can say that the vagina's acidic environment is a direct consequence of the estrogen circulating levels. As seen above, estrogen levels are influenced, among others, by the gut microbiome.

2. The Microbiome and Cancer Development

Many factors promote a healthy flora versus dysbiosis, usually promoting functioning cells versus cancer. In a considerable measure, these factors are the same. In other words, the factors associated with an unhealthy gut or vaginal flora are the ones that are also associated with cancer. Some of the factors associated with dysbiosis and cancer are low socioeconomic status, ethnicity, poor access to medical care, a high prevalence of sexually transmitted diseases, smoking, alcohol consumption, obesity, reduced physical activity, metabolic syndrome, high levels of stress, aging, hormonal imbalances, genetic and epigenetic factors, impaired immunity, the human papillomavirus [22,23]. Smoking, douching, and obesity were all linked to bacterial vaginosis [2].

Changes in the microbiome also induce complex changes in human cells [24]. From a biological perspective, the normal cervicovaginal microbiome is composed mainly of *Lactobacillus* spp., thus exhibiting low bacterial diversity and protecting against carcinogenesis through various mechanisms [25]. The lactobacilli secrete lactic acid, and the low vaginal pH promotes healthy local homeostasis. The lactobacilli also secrete cytokines, antimicrobial peptides, and other metabolites that protect the local epithelium. They promote a healthy level of physiological inflammation that stimulates the immune system to fight against pathogens.

On the other hand, the dysbiotic cervicovaginal microbiome exhibits a high diversity of microorganisms, primarily obligate and strict anaerobes, that lead to a high vaginal pH. The bacteria promote the disruption of the epithelial barrier and secrete various metabolites and enzymes such as sialidase, proinflammatory cytokines and chemokines, reactive oxygen species, and other carcinogenic metabolites that lead to chronic inflammation and a dysregulated local metabolism. Further down the line, they also lead to genotoxicity and genomic instability, as well as altered proliferation and altered apoptosis. The dysbiotic environment also promotes angiogenesis. The chronic inflammation activates immune cells that secrete even more proinflammatory cytokines and chemokines such as Interleukin (IL)-6, IL-8 or Tumor necrosis factor (TNF), resulting in even more reactive oxygen species that further promote carcinogenic mechanisms. Hence, there are many different mechanisms through which the microbiota can impact carcinogenesis [25–27].

2.1. The Microbiome and Endometrial Cancer

Whereas the most common gynecological cancer in developing countries is cervical cancer, because of high rates of Human Papilloma Virus (HPV) infection and low rates of vaccination, the most common gynecological cancer in developed countries is endometrial cancer [2]. Many factors are associated with endometrial cancer, including high estrogen levels, obesity, chronic inflammation, and post-menopausal hormonal therapy.

The gut microbiome and the circulating estrogen levels are intensively connected as a feedback loop, influencing each other. We can hypothesize that the gut microbiome, the estrobolome in particular, has a part to play in the development of endometrial cancer, but more research is needed. Moreover, estrogen metabolism and the gut and vaginal microbiome are influenced by obesity. There is an association between the body mass index, the estrogen metabolism and the composition of the vaginal and gut microbiome [2,28].

A high vaginal pH is correlated with endometrial cancer, usually due to a disbalance of the vaginal flora. For instance, recent studies showed that *Atopobium vaginae* and *Porphyromonas* among other bacteria that raise the vaginal pH are more prevalent in the vaginal flora of women with endometrial hyperplasia or endometrial cancer [29]. It is believed that this promotes chronic endometrial inflammation that turns on the carcinogenesis process [2].

Compared with benign uterine lesions, endometrial cancer is associated with a decrease in the diversity of the local endometrial microbiota [30]. Some less-represented endometrial carcinoma species are *Salinibacter ruber*, *Bacillus tropicus*, *Pusillimonas* sp., *Riemerella anatipestifer*, *Nostocales cyanobacterium* HT-58-2 and *Corynebacterium pseudotuberculosis* [31]. This leads to an overgrowth of the remaining species. Micrococcus overgrowth is associated with an inflammatory profile in endometrial cancer, with increased IL-6 and IL-17 mRNA levels. *Bilophila*, *Rheinheimera*, *Rhodobacter*, *Vogesella* and *Megamonas* are overgrown in benign uterine lesions [30]. *Atopobium vaginae* and *Popayromonas somerae* induce the production of proinflammatory cytokines IL-1α, IL-1β, IL-17α, and TNFα; they also alter the transcription of CCL13, CCL8, CXCL2, IL22 and IL9 [32]. The production of IL-17α induces the production of IL-8 and TNFα, which are promoting factors for endometrial cell proliferation and angiogenesis [33]. TNFα also contributes to resistance to chemotherapy and metastasis development [34]. In endometrial cancer, IL1α and IL1β are overexpressed and promote cell proliferation, adhesion, invasion, and angiogenesis [35].

2.2. The Microbiome and Ovarian Cancer

Ovarian cancer is a relatively rare tumor with a bad prognosis since it develops inconspicuously with no symptoms until the late stages.

Genital dysbiosis has been associated with ovarian cancer, although more research is needed to draw causality conclusions [36]. Sexually transmitted bacteria such as *Chlamydia* spp. and *Mycoplasma* spp. that cause chronic reproductive tract inflammation have been associated with ovarian cancer. For instance, more than 60% of ovarian tumors contain such intracellular bacteria [2]. Other microorganisms associated with ovarian cancer are *Proteobacteria*, *Acinetobacter* spp., *Brucella* and even viruses such as cytomegalovirus or HPV [2,37,38].

Lactobacilli species in the cervicovaginal part of the genital tract have a protective role against ovarian cancer [39]. BRCA mutation carriers are associated with a reduction in *Lactobacillus* spp. This association is more substantial in younger patients [40].

An increase in *Proteobacteria* and *Fusobacteria* characterizes the microbiome in the tumor tissue compared to normal tissue; these gram-negative bacteria make the microbiome more immunogenic [41–43].

Pelvic inflammatory disease is a risk factor for ovarian cancer [2,44–46]. Bacterial flagellin and lipopolysaccharide (LPS) have an essential role in driving inflammation in ovarian cancer by inducing a response in pattern recognition receptors TLR2, 4, and 5 [41,47–54], leading to activation of NF-kappa B signaling [42]. LPS stimulate cancer cells inducing PI3K activation, EMT and overexpression of Vimentin, Snail, α-SMA, TCF, MMP2, N-cadherin, Slug, and MMP9 [53]. Even though LPS activates tumoral-associated macrophages, pushing them towards the M1 profile [55,56] and making them cytotoxic and cytostatic for ovarian cancer cells [57], a recent study has shown that administration of LPS does not prolong and may even shorten survival [58].

The increase in Gram-negative bacteria leads to an increase in lysophospholipids, which are by-products of bacterial metabolism [59,60]. Lysophosphatids are similar to lysophospholipids; in ovarian cancer patients, lysophosphatids plasma levels are increased [61,62]. In ovarian cancer cells, lysophosphatidic acid can increase the expression of angiogenesis promoters [63] and induce cell migration, invasion and proliferation [64–70]. A short description of bacterial metabolites effects on ovarian cancer is displayed in Table 1.

Bacteria metabolize tryptophan, producing indole-derivatives [71–76], which act on the aryl hydrocarbon and pregnane X receptors [77–79]. Aryl hydrocarbon receptor is involved in immune regulation [76,80]. Tryptophan rich diet leads to the proliferation of Lactobacilli [77], which prevents the proliferation of pathogenic bacteria [77,81–83]. Tryptophan and indolepropionic acid levels are reduced in the serum of ovarian cancer patients [84–88] and are inversely correlated with the stage of the disease [88].

Antibiotics (glycylcyclines, erythromycins, tetracyclines and chloramphenicol) can block cellular proliferation and reduce the proportion of ovarian stem cells [89]. Minocycline [90–93], Ciprofloxacin [94], and Salinomycin [87,95–100] can reduce the proliferation rate of ovarian cancer cells. In murine models, antibiotics can also be used to prevent cisplatin resistance [101], and minocycline can potentiate the activity of topoisomerase inhibitors [102].

Even though many studies suggest a potential benefit of antibiotic therapy, there is a study in which the treatment of mice grafted with ovarian cancer with neomycin, ampicillin, vancomycin, and metronidazole was associated with increased invasiveness and growth of the grafts [103].

Table 1. Effects of bacterial metabolites on ovarian cancer.

Bacterial Flagellin	Activation of NF-kappa B Signaling [42]
Lipopolysaccharides	PI3K activation, EMT, overexpression of Vimentin, Snail, α-SMA, TCF, MMP2, N-cadherin, Slug, and MMP9 activation tumoral-associated macrophages [53]
Lysophosphatids	angiogenesis, cell migration, invasion and proliferation [61,62]
Indole-derivatives	immune regulation [76,80]

2.3. The Microbiome and Cervical Cancer

Cervical cancer is a common malignancy in women, especially in developing countries where the HPV vaccination rate is low. Over 99% of cervical cancer biopsies contain HPV Deoxyribonucleic acid (DNA) as determined by Polymerase chain reaction (PCR) [2,104]. HPV is the major carcinogenic factor in the evolution of cervical cancer through the expression of E6 and E7 proteins. The most high-risk genotypes are HPV 16 and HPV 18. However, it is essential to note that 85–90% of HPV infections with high-risk genotypes are spontaneously cleared [2]. The high-risk HPV infections that persist can, in time, lead to cervical intraepithelial neoplasia (CIN)—low grade and then high grade—and then progress to invasive cervical cancer.

The link between vaginal dysbiosis and HPV persistence and neoplastic transformation is yet to be established. Still, various studies have already shown that the composition of the cervicovaginal flora differs in women with different HPV statuses [105,106]. HPV persistence has been linked with bacterial vaginosis by various studies, and anaerobic flora is conducive to HPV persistence [2,105–107]. A high vaginal bacterial diversity and a depletion of *Lactobacillus* spp. have been repeatedly associated with a low clearance of HPV.

HPV-negative women have been shown to host mainly *Lactobacillus crispatus* and *Lactobacillus iners*. However, HPV-positive women with a normal cervix contain the two lactobacillus species in different proportions. The risk of cervical transformation is higher with *Lactobacillus iners* than with *Lactobacillus crispatus* [108]. Once the HPV infection progresses toward cervical intraepithelial neoplasia, the cervicovaginal bacterial diversity increases correspondingly. The *Lactobacillus* spp is depleted, and the vaginal pH is elevated. The highest diversity is found in invasive cervical cancer (*Fusobacterium necrophorum*, *Gardnerella vaginalis*, *Sneathia* etc.) [2,108,109].

Various studies have shown that vaginal *Sneathia* associates with HPV persistence and pathological progression to cancer. *Atopobium* spp. is also associated with HPV persistence [110].

Other organisms that have been shown to influence the transformation of HPV lesions are *Candida albicans, Chlamydia trachomatis* and *Ureaplasma urealyticum* [2].

The increase in the diversity of the microbial flora leads to the production of cytokines which amplify the inflammatory response [108,111–113], leading to immune dysregulation in the reproductive tract and thus creating a more suitable site for tumor development [24].

Mycoplasma genitalium causes bacterial cervicitis and vaginitis, increasing the incidence of cervical lesions [114,115]. *Chlamydia trachomatis* damages the cervical mucosa and promotes infection of the cervical epithelium by HPV [116,117]. See Table 2 below.

Table 2. Examples of bacteria associated with female reproductive tract pathology.

Bacteria found to be associated with female reproductive tract pathology, including cancer	*Popayromonar somerae, Chlamydia* spp., *Mycoplasma* spp., Proteobacteria, *Acinetobacter* spp., *Brucella* spp., *Fusobacterium necrophorum, Gardnerella vaginalis, Sneathia* spp., *Candida albicans, Chlamydia trachomatis, Ureaplasma urealyticum*	
Examples of how bacteria might induce pathologic changes in the female reproductive tract	*Mycoplasma genitalium*	Cervicitis and vaginitis, chromosomal lesions [114,115]
	Chlamydiatrachomatis	Increased risk of infection of the cervical epithelium by HPV [116,117]
	Fusobacterium spp.	Increased production of IL-4, IL-10 and TGF-b1 [118]

Fusobacterium leads to increased production of interleukin-4, interleukin-10 and TGF-beta1 in the cervix and vagina; these cytokines are also increased in cervical cancer and squamous intraepithelial disease [118].

3. Interaction between Cancer Treatment and the Microbiome

The main pillars of cancer treatment are surgery, radiotherapy, chemotherapy, targeted molecules, and immunotherapy. This part of the article explores the interaction between cancer treatment and the microbiome. We will summarize what is known on the female reproductive tract microbiome, and in addition we will also explore the gut microbiome. The gut microbiome is much more investigated, and we hope that these insights will lead to new interesting research projects on the female reproductive tract microbiome as well.

Moreover, understanding the gut microbiome is important because a lack of oestrogen-metabolizing bacteria (from a lower diversity of the gut microbiota after chemotherapy for instance) could influence the vaginal microbiome composition. Therefore, strategies targeted towards the gut microbiome might have an indirect effect on the vaginal microbiome as well.

It is well-known that both radiotherapy and chemotherapy can cause gut mucositis and diarrhea. They also decrease the diversity of the gut microbiome, which is usually linked to digestive tract side effects. In contrast, radiotherapy and chemotherapy seem to increase bacterial diversity of the female reproductive tract, and increased bacterial diversity is a sign of disease, as previously explained.

Immunotherapy has emerged as a treatment in multiple types of cancer in recent years. Regarding gynecological cancers, it is of interest especially in patients with MSI-H endometrial, cervical, and ovarian cancer. Not much is yet known about the effects of immunotherapy such as Nivolumab, Ipilimumab and Pembrolizumab on microbiomes. However, we can hypothesize that there is an interesting interplay between immunotherapy and microbiomes since they both act on and modulate the immune system. More research is needed in this direction.

Some specific bacteria-like microorganisms, such as *Bifidobacterium longum*, Ruminococcaceae and *Akkermansia muciniphila* were found to be more abundant in fecal samples collected from PD-1-responding patients. Oral supplementation with *Akkermansia muciniphila* proved beneficial in restoring response to immunotherapy in mouse models of epithelial tumors. The authors noticed an increase in the recruitment of CCR9+, CXCR3+, CD4+ T lymphocytes [119]. Proposed mechanisms involve the production of short-chain fatty acids and their pro-apoptotic role in cancer cells through activation of p21 cell cycle inhibitor and specific caspases, but also activation of the mTOR-S6K and STAT3 pathways in T-cells [120]. Administration of an oral cocktail of live Bifidobacterium to tumor-bearing mice significantly improved tumor control for several weeks. The same mice presented elevated levels of tumor-specific T cells in the periphery and antigen-specific CD8+ T cells within the tumor. Authors noticed a lack of anti-tumor effect in immunodeficient mice or mice treated with previously heat-inactivated Bifidobacterium [121]. Opposite results come from the study of Kim et al., who expanded on parabiotics as non-viable microbial cells in the form of heat-killed Bifidobacterium or Lactobacillus. These strains induced apoptosis of human colorectal carcinoma RKO cells in vitro and also revealed anti-tumor effects in an RKO cell-derived xenograft model through the activation of caspase-9, 3, 7 and PARP [122].

Interestingly, antibiotics seem to decrease immunotherapy's efficacy, suggesting a link between these novel treatments and the microbiomes. Antibiotics also seem to increase the toxicity of chemotherapy. Moreover, radiotherapy, chemotherapy and immunotherapy are all less efficient in a germ-free mouse; fecal-matter transplantation and probiotics have been shown to improve the efficacy of immunotherapy [2,123–126].

The gut microbiota may be involved in the prevention of chemotherapy-associated toxicity, improved efficacy of oncologic treatment, prevention of surgical morbidity, and quality of life. Diarrhea, abdominal pain, vomiting, and weight loss are critical adverse reactions to chemotherapy that cause significant morbidity. Preventive intervention on the gut microbiota can influence the pathogenesis of mucositis through TLR2 signaling, mediation of vitamin B production, and microbial enzymatic degradation. Additionally, prognostic markers can be derived from specific microbiota patterns. The bowel mucosa load with *Fusobacterium nucleatum* strains correlates with worse prognostic in patients with colorectal cancer [125].

Modulating microbiomes had essential health benefits in many chronic and inflammatory diseases, including irritable bowel syndrome and recurring *Clostridioides difficile* infections and implications in cancer prevention and response to treatment.

Gut microbiota modulation is represented by probiotics, prebiotics, antibiotics or other drugs, or microbiota transplantation [127].

Bifidobacterium and Bacteroides species have been associated with immune modulation and estrogen metabolism and are under investigation for preventing estrogen-derived cancer such as breast, endometrial, and ovarian cancer [2]. Probiotics containing *Lactobacillus lactis* engineered to secrete an antimicrobial peptide involved in gut homeostasis (pancreatitis-associated protein) proved to reduce enteritis induced by 5-Fluorouracil in cancer patients. The mechanism was represented by a reduced abundance of pathogenic bacteria such as *Enterobacteriaceae* in the intestine, thus reducing the intensity of mucositis [128]

Fecal microbiota transplantation reduced the side effects generated by chemotherapy and radiotherapy [129]. However, the most important studies are related to fecal microbiota transplantation from responders to germ-free mice with xenograft tumors (melanoma, lung or kidney) which showed an increased response to checkpoint inhibitors [130].

Approaches for modulating vaginal microbiomes are under investigation. They aim to modify vaginal microbiota to optimal Lactobacillus-dominant flora to prevent carcinogenesis and in cancer patients to increase the effectiveness of treatments and decrease toxicity. Novel antimicrobials and probiotics such as intravaginally delivered vaginal lactobacilli formulations, biofilm disruptors, and vaginal microbiota transplantation are being considered.

Vaginal probiotic lactobacilli (*L. crispatus* strain CTV-05 known as LACTIN- V) have been tested with success in clinical trials, mainly for the treatment of bacterial vaginosis or urinary tract infection (UTI) [131,132].

Vaginal microbiota transplantation (VMT) from donors with optimal vaginal flora is a novel potential treatment option under investigation for women with vaginal disorders.

However, there is an unknown long-term risk of microbiome transplants (fecal or vaginal) related to the potential transfer of antimicrobial-resistant microorganisms, which may be problematic in immunodepleted cancer patients.

Probiotics consisting of *Lactobacillus* spp. might aid in the treatment of cervicovaginal dysbiosis and persistent HPV infections [133,134]. *Lactobacillus* spp. probiotics might increase the clearance of HPV when used long-term in certain patients [134,135]. Since it is well established that persistent HPV infections increase the risk of cervical cancer, *Lactobacillus* spp. probiotics might be considered in HPV positive patients. However, more research is needed before establishing clear links and then guidelines.

A study conducted by Tsementzi et al. showed that radiation therapy alone in post-menopausal patients with gynaecologic cancer leads to a perturbation of the vaginal microbiome with a decrease of *Lactobacillus* spp. The study showed a higher vaginal bacterial diversity in cancer patients with respect to healthy patients and a higher vaginal bacterial diversity in post-radiotherapy with respect to pre-radiotherapy. This might be associated with some post-radiotherapy symptoms in patients with vulvovaginal atrophy and these findings might have implications for future therapeutic interventions, such as probiotics or vaginal microbiome transplantation [136].

Overall, not much is known about the female reproductive tract microbiome and its changes during cancer treatment, and even less is known on the influence of the female reproductive microbiome on the response to various treatments.

4. The Microbiome and Endometriosis

Endometriosis is a multifactorial disease whose etiology is not entirely established. One theory is "retrograde menstruation" where the menstrual flux and viable endometrial cells go through the fallopian tubes to the peritoneum, where they adhere. There is an essential component of inflammation, but it is not yet clear if this is a cause or an effect of endometriosis. Interestingly, the composition of the gut microbiome is also linked to this disease. A healthy gut is composed of a balanced distribution of *Firmicutes* spp. and *Bacteroidetes* spp. However, in endometriosis, this balance is altered with a predominance of either one or the other species. Endometriosis development can induce a change in the gut microbiome [137,138]. The complex interrelation between endometriosis, circulating estrogen levels, and gut bacteria warrants further research.

5. Conclusions

The microbiome, in general, and the female reproductive tract microbiome, is an exciting research avenue. More and more studies show a connection between different microbiome compositions and various cancers. There is a low diversity of bacterial species in the vagina and cervix, represented mainly by *Lactobacillus* spp. which prevents colonization of the female genital tract with pathogenic bacteria. The proliferation of pathogenic bacteria leads to a higher diversity of the microbiome. This abnormally diverse microbiome can modulate the immune response in the female genital tract creating an environment characterized by chronic inflammation, which is favorable for developing neoplasia. Some products of bacterial metabolism have carcinogenic properties and act upon the normal cells of the genital tract leading to genetic alterations. Other products of bacterial metabolism have angiogenic properties and promote neovascularization, which favors vascular invasion and metastasis.

Moreover, the microbiome also seems to influence the response to therapy and toxicity. The estrobolome, through its effect on estrogen circulating levels, can impact both the composition of the cervicovaginal microbiome and carcinogenesis. More research is needed to describe these interactions better and find ways of harnessing this information toward better treatments.

Author Contributions: Conceptualization, O.G.T. and R.A.T.; methodology, O.G.T. and D.M.B.; software, L.V.; validation, R.I.M., L.N.G. and G.L.S.; investigation, L.V. and S.A.M.; resources, R.A.T. and B.C.T.; writing—original draft preparation, O.G.T. and D.M.B.; writing—review and editing, R.I.M., D.M.B. and L.V.; visualization, L.N.G.; supervision, R.M.A.; funding acquisition, G.L.S. All authors have read and agreed to the published version of the manuscript.

Funding: Publication of this paper was supported by the University of Medicine and Pharmacy "Carol Davila", through the institutional program "Publish not Perish".

Institutional Review Board Statement: Not applicable.

Informed Consent Statement: Not applicable.

Conflicts of Interest: The authors declare no conflict of interest.

References

1. Marchesi, J.R.; Ravel, J. The vocabulary of microbiome research: A proposal. *Microbiome* **2015**, *3*, 31. [CrossRef] [PubMed]
2. Aniewski, P.; Ilhan, Z.E.; Herbst-Kralovetz, M.M. The microbiome and gynaecological cancer development, prevention and therapy. *Nat. Rev. Urol.* **2020**, *17*, 232–250. [CrossRef] [PubMed]
3. Baker, J.M.; Chase, D.M.; Herbst-Kralovetz, M.M. Uterine Microbiota: Residents, Tourists, or Invaders? *Front. Immunol.* **2018**, *9*, 208. [CrossRef] [PubMed]
4. Huttenhower, C.; Gevers, D.; Knight, R.; Abubucker, S.; Badger, J.H.; Chinwalla, A.T.; Creasy, H.H.; Earl, A.M.; FitzGerald, M.G.; Fulton, R.S.; et al. Structure, function and diversity of the healthy human microbiome. *Nature* **2012**, *486*, 207–214.
5. Lynch, S.V.; Pedersen, O. The Human Intestinal Microbiome in Health and Disease. *N. Engl. J. Med.* **2016**, *375*, 2369–2379. [CrossRef]
6. Sepich-Poore, G.D.; Zitvogel, L.; Straussman, R.; Hasty, J.; Wargo, J.A.; Knight, R. The microbiome and human cancer. *Science* **2021**, *371*, eabc4552. [CrossRef]
7. Miller, E.; Beasley, D.; Dunn, R.; Archie, E. Lactobacilli Dominance and Vaginal pH: Why is the Human Vaginal Microbiome Unique? *Front. Microbiol.* **2016**, *7*, 1936. [CrossRef]
8. Nunn, K.L.; Forney, L.J. Unraveling the Dynamics of the Human Vaginal Microbiome. *Yale J. Biol. Med.* **2016**, *89*, 331–337.
9. Gajer, P.; Brotman, R.M.; Bai, G.; Sakamoto, J.; Schütte, U.M.E.; Zhong, X.; Koenig, S.S.K.; Fu, L.; Ma, Z.; Zhou, X.; et al. Temporal Dynamics of the Human Vaginal Microbiota. *Sci. Transl. Med.* **2012**, *4*, 132ra52. [CrossRef]
10. Witkin, S.S.; Mendes-Soares, H.; Linhares, I.M.; Jayaram, A.; Ledger, W.J.; Forney, L.J. Influence of Vaginal Bacteria and d- and l-Lactic Acid Isomers on Vaginal Extracellular Matrix Metalloproteinase Inducer: Implications for Protection against Upper Genital Tract Infections. *mBio* **2013**, *4*, e00460-13. [CrossRef]
11. Antonio, M.A.D.; Rabe, L.K.; Hillier, S.L. Colonization of the Rectum by *Lactobacillus* Species and Decreased Risk of Bacterial Vaginosis. *J. Infect. Dis.* **2005**, *192*, 394–398. [CrossRef] [PubMed]
12. Flores, R.; Shi, J.; Fuhrman, B.; Xu, X.; Veenstra, T.D.; Gail, M.H.; Gajer, P.; Ravel, J.; Goedert, J.J. Fecal microbial determinants of fecal and systemic estrogens and estrogen metabolites: A cross-sectional study. *J. Transl. Med.* **2012**, *10*, 253. [CrossRef]
13. Baker, J.M.; Al-Nakkash, L.; Herbst-Kralovetz, M.M. Estrogen–gut microbiome axis: Physiological and clinical implications. *Maturitas* **2017**, *103*, 45–53. [CrossRef] [PubMed]
14. McIntosh, F.M.; Maison, N.; Holtrop, G.; Young, P.; Stevens, V.J.; Ince, J.; Johnstone, A.M.; Lobley, G.E.; Flint, H.J.; Louis, P. Phylogenetic distribution of genes encoding β-glucuronidase activity in human colonic bacteria and the impact of diet on faecal glycosidase activities. *Environ. Microbiol.* **2012**, *14*, 1876–1887. [CrossRef] [PubMed]
15. Gloux, K.; Berteau, O.; El Oumami, H.; Béguet, F.; Leclerc, M.; Doré, J. A metagenomic -glucuronidase uncovers a core adaptive function of the human intestinal microbiome. *Proc. Natl. Acad. Sci. USA* **2011**, *108* (Suppl. S1), 4539–4546. [CrossRef]
16. Komorowski, A.S.; Pezo, R.C. Untapped "-omics": The microbial metagenome, estrobolome, and their influence on the development of breast cancer and response to treatment. *Breast Cancer Res. Treat.* **2019**, *179*, 287–300. [CrossRef]
17. Tilg, H.; Marchesi, J.R. Too much fat for the gut's microbiota. *Gut* **2012**, *61*, 474–475. [CrossRef]
18. Goedert, J.J.; Jones, G.; Hua, X.; Xu, X.; Yu, G.; Flores, R.; Falk, R.T.; Gail, M.H.; Shi, J.; Ravel, J.; et al. Investigation of the Association Between the Fecal Microbiota and Breast Cancer in Postmenopausal Women: A Population-Based Case-Control Pilot Study. *Gynecol. Oncol.* **2015**, *107*, djv147. [CrossRef]
19. AlHilli, M.M.; Bae-Jump, V. Diet and gut microbiome interactions in gynecologic cancer. *Gynecol. Oncol.* **2020**, *159*, 299–308. [CrossRef]
20. Muhleisen, A.L.; Herbst-Kralovetz, M.M. Menopause and the vaginal microbiome. *Maturitas* **2016**, *91*, 42–50. [CrossRef]
21. Mirmonsef, P.; Hotton, A.L.; Gilbert, D.; Gioia, C.J.; Maric, D.; Hope, T.J.; Landay, A.L.; Spear, G.T. Glycogen Levels in Undiluted Genital Fluid and Their Relationship to Vaginal pH, Estrogen, and Progesterone. *PLoS ONE* **2016**, *11*, e0153553. [CrossRef] [PubMed]
22. Lewis, F.M.T.; Bernstein, K.T.P.; Aral, S.O.P. Vaginal Microbiome and Its Relationship to Behavior, Sexual Health, and Sexually Transmitted Diseases. *Obstet. Gynecol.* **2017**, *129*, 643–654. [CrossRef] [PubMed]

23. Martin, D.H.; Marrazzo, J.M. The Vaginal Microbiome: Current Understanding and Future Directions. *J. Infect. Dis.* **2016**, *214* (Suppl. S1), S36–S41. [CrossRef] [PubMed]
24. Schwabe, R.F.; Jobin, C. The microbiome and cancer. *Nat. Rev. Cancer.* **2013**, *13*, 800–812. [CrossRef]
25. Garrett, W.S. Cancer and the microbiota. *Science* **2015**, *348*, 80–86. [CrossRef]
26. Rajagopala, S.V.; Vashee, S.; Oldfield, L.M.; Suzuki, Y.; Venter, J.C.; Telenti, A.; Nelson, K.E. The Human Microbiome and Cancer. *Cancer Prev. Res.* **2017**, *10*, 226–234. [CrossRef]
27. Dzutsev, A.; Goldszmid, R.S.; Viaud, S.; Zitvogel, L.; Trinchieri, G. The role of the microbiota in inflammation, carcinogenesis, and cancer therapy. *Eur. J. Immunol.* **2014**, *45*, 17–31. [CrossRef]
28. Tilg, H.; Moschen, A.R.; Kaser, A. Obesity and the microbiota. *Gastroenterology* **2009**, *136*, 1476–1483. [CrossRef]
29. Walther-António, M.R.S.; Chen, J.; Multinu, F.; Hokenstad, A.; Distad, T.J.; Cheek, E.H.; Keeney, G.L.; Creedon, D.J.; Nelson, H.; Mariani, A.; et al. Potential contribution of the uterine microbiome in the development of endometrial cancer. *Genome Med.* **2016**, *8*, 1–15. [CrossRef]
30. Lu, W.; He, F.; Lin, Z.; Liu, S.; Tang, L.; Huang, Y.; Hu, Z. Dysbiosis of the endometrial microbiota and its association with inflammatory cytokines in endometrial cancer. *Int. J. Cancer.* **2021**, *148*, 1708–1716. [CrossRef]
31. Gonzalez-Bosquet, J.; Pedra-Nobre, S.; Devor, E.; Thiel, K.; Goodheart, M.; Bender, D.; Leslie, K. Bacterial, Archaea, and Viral Transcripts (BAVT) Expression in Gynecological Cancers and Correlation with Regulatory Regions of the Genome. *Cancers* **2021**, *13*, 1109. [CrossRef] [PubMed]
32. Caselli, E.; Soffritti, I.; D'Accolti, M.; Piva, I.; Greco, P.; Bonaccorsi, G. Atopobium Vaginae and Porphyromonas Somerae Induce Proinflammatory Cytokines Expression in Endometrial Cells: A Possible Implication for Endometrial Cancer? *Cancer Manag. Res.* **2019**, *11*, 8571–8575. [CrossRef] [PubMed]
33. Hirata, T.; Osuga, Y.; Hamasaki, K.; Yoshino, O.; Ito, M.; Hasegawa, A.; Takemura, Y.; Hirota, Y.; Nose, E.; Morimoto, C.; et al. Interleukin (IL)-17A Stimulates IL-8 Secretion, Cyclooxygenase-2 Expression, and Cell Proliferation of Endometriotic Stromal Cells. *Endocrinology* **2007**, *149*, 1260–1267. [CrossRef] [PubMed]
34. Smith, H.O.; Stephens, N.D.; Qualls, C.R.; Fligelman, T.; Wang, T.; Lin, C.-Y.; Burton, E.H.; Griffith, J.K.; Pollard, J.W. The clinical significance of inflammatory cytokines in primary cell culture in endometrial carcinoma. *Mol. Oncol.* **2012**, *7*, 41–54. [CrossRef] [PubMed]
35. Keita, M.; Bessette, P.; Pelmus, M.; Ainmelk, Y.; Aris, A. Expression of interleukin-1 (IL-1) ligands system in the most common endometriosis-associated ovarian cancer subtypes. *J. Ovarian Res.* **2010**, *3*, 3–8. [CrossRef]
36. Li, H.; Zang, Y.; Wang, C.; Li, H.; Fan, A.; Han, C.; Xue, F. The Interaction Between Microorganisms, Metabolites, and Immune System in the Female Genital Tract Microenvironment. *Front. Cell. Infect. Microbiol.* **2020**, *10*, 796. [CrossRef]
37. Banerjee, S.; Tian, T.; Wei, Z.; Shih, N.; Feldman, M.D.; Alwine, J.C.; Coukos, G.; Robertson, E.S. The ovarian cancer oncobiome. *Oncotarget* **2017**, *8*, 36225–36245. [CrossRef]
38. Shanmughapriya, S.; Senthilkumar, G.; Vinodhini, K.; Das, B.C.; Vasanthi, N.; Natarajaseenivasan, K. Viral and bacterial aetiologies of epithelial ovarian cancer. *Eur. J. Clin. Microbiol. Infect. Dis.* **2012**, *31*, 2311–2317. [CrossRef]
39. Xu, J.; Peng, J.J.; Yang, W.; Fu, K.; Zhang, Y. Vaginal microbiomes and ovarian cancer: A review. *Am. J. Cancer Res.* **2020**, *10*, 743–756.
40. Nené, N.R.; Reisel, D.; Leimbach, A.; Franchi, D.; Jones, A.; Evans, I.; Knapp, S.; Ryan, A.; Ghazali, S.; Timms, J.F.; et al. Association between the cervicovaginal microbiome, BRCA1 mutation status, and risk of ovarian cancer: A case-control study. *Lancet Oncol.* **2019**, *20*, 1171–1182. [CrossRef]
41. Wang, Q.; Zhao, L.; Han, L.; Fu, G.; Tuo, X.; Ma, S.; Li, Q.; Wang, Y.; Liang, D.; Tang, M.; et al. The differential distribution of bacteria between cancerous and noncancerous ovarian tissues in situ. *J Ovarian Res.* **2020**, *13*, 8. [CrossRef] [PubMed]
42. Zhou, B.; Sun, C.; Huang, J.; Xia, M.; Guo, E.; Li, N.; Lu, H.; Shan, W.; Wu, Y.; Li, Y.; et al. The biodiversity Composition of Microbiome in Ovarian Carcinoma Patients. *Sci. Rep.* **2019**, *9*, 1–11. [CrossRef] [PubMed]
43. Poore, G.D.; Kopylova, E.; Zhu, Q.; Carpenter, C.; Fraraccio, S.; Wandro, S.; Kosciolek, T.; Janssen, S.; Metcalf, J.; Song, S.J.; et al. Microbiome analyses of blood and tissues suggest cancer diagnostic approach. *Nature* **2020**, *579*, 567–574. [CrossRef] [PubMed]
44. Rasmussen, C.B.; Kjaer, S.K.; Albieri, V.; Bandera, E.V.; Doherty, J.A.; Høgdall, E.; Webb, P.M.; Jordan, S.J.; Rossing, M.A.; Wicklund, K.G.; et al. Pelvic Inflammatory Disease and the Risk of Ovarian Cancer and Borderline Ovarian Tumors: A Pooled Analysis of 13 Case-Control Studies. *Am. J. Epidemiol.* **2016**, *185*, 8–20. [CrossRef] [PubMed]
45. Rasmussen, C.B.; Faber, M.T.; Jensen, A.; Høgdall, E.; Høgdall, C.; Blaakær, J.; Kjaer, S.K. Pelvic inflammatory disease and risk of invasive ovarian cancer and ovarian borderline tumors. *Cancer Causes Control.* **2013**, *24*, 1459–1464. [CrossRef]
46. Mert, I.; Walther-Antonio, M.; Mariani, A. Case for a role of the microbiome in gynecologic cancers: Clinician's perspective. *J. Obstet. Gynaecol. Res.* **2018**, *44*, 1693–1704. [CrossRef]
47. Rutkowski, M.R.; Stephen, T.L.; Svoronos, N.; Allegrezza, M.J.; Tesone, A.J.; Perales-Puchalt, A.; Brencicova, E.; Escovar-Fadul, X.; Nguyen, J.M.; Cadungog, M.G.; et al. Microbially Driven TLR5-Dependent Signaling Governs Distal Malignant Progression through Tumor-Promoting Inflammation. *Cancer Cell* **2014**, *27*, 27–40. [CrossRef]
48. Wang, Y.; Sun, L.; Chen, S.; Guo, S.; Yue, T.; Hou, Q.; Feng, M.; Xu, H.; Liu, Y.; Wang, P.; et al. The administration of Escherichia coli Nissle 1917 ameliorates irinotecan–induced intestinal barrier dysfunction and gut microbial dysbiosis in mice. *Life Sci.* **2019**, *231*, 116529. [CrossRef]

49. Kashani, B.; Zandi, Z.; Bashash, D.; Zaghal, A.; Momeny, M.; Poursani, E.M.; Pourbagheri-Sigaroodi, A.; Mousavi, S.A.; Ghaffari, S.H. Small molecule inhibitor of TLR4 inhibits ovarian cancer cell proliferation: New insight into the anticancer effect of TAK-242 (Resatorvid). *Cancer Chemother. Pharmacol.* **2019**, *85*, 47–59. [CrossRef]
50. Kelly, M.G.; Alvero, A.B.; Chen, R.; Silasi, D.-A.; Abrahams, V.M.; Chan, S.; Visintin, I.; Rutherford, T.; Mor, G. TLR-4 Signaling Promotes Tumor Growth and Paclitaxel Chemoresistance in Ovarian Cancer. *Cancer Res* **2006**, *66*, 3859–3868. [CrossRef]
51. Glezerman, M.; Mazot, M.; Maymon, E.; Piura, B.; Prinsloo, I.; Benharroch, D.; Yanai-Inbar, I.; Huleihel, M. Tumor necrosis factor-alpha and interleukin-6 are differently expressed by fresh human cancerous ovarian tissue and primary cell lines. *Eur. Cytokine Netw.* **1998**, *9*, 171–179. [PubMed]
52. Huleihel, M.; Maymon, E.; Piura, B.; Prinsloo, I.; Benharroch, D.; Yanai-Inbar, I.; Glezerman, M. Distinct patterns of expression of interleukin-1 alpha and beta by normal and cancerous human ovarian tissues. *Eur. Cytokine Netw.* **1997**, *8*, 179–187. [PubMed]
53. Bin Park, G.; Chung, Y.H.; Kim, D. Induction of galectin-1 by TLR-dependent PI3K activation enhances epithelial-mesenchymal transition of metastatic ovarian cancer cells. *Oncol. Rep.* **2017**, *37*, 3137–3145. [CrossRef] [PubMed]
54. Muccioli, M.; Benencia, F. Toll-like receptors in ovarian cancer as targets for immunotherapies. *Front. Immunol.* **2014**, *5*, 341. [CrossRef] [PubMed]
55. Trenti, A.; Boscaro, C.; Tedesco, S.; Cignarella, A.; Trevisi, L.; Bolego, C. Effects of digitoxin on cell migration in ovarian cancer inflammatory microenvironment. *Biochem. Pharmacol.* **2018**, *154*, 414–423. [CrossRef]
56. Wanderley, C.W.; Colón, D.F.; Luiz, J.P.M.; Oliveira, F.F.; Viacava, P.R.; Leite, C.A.; Pereira, J.A.; Silva, C.M.; Silva, C.R.; Silva, R.L.; et al. Paclitaxel reduces tumor growth by reprogramming tumor-associated macrophages to an M1- profile in a TLR4-dependent manner. *Cancer Res.* **2018**, *78*, 5891–5900. [CrossRef]
57. Han, X.; Wilbanks, G.D.; Devaja, O.; Ruperelia, V.; Raju, K.S. IL-2 enhances standard IFNgamma/LPS activation of macrophage cytotoxicity to human ovarian carcinoma in vitro: A potential for adoptive cellular immunotherapy. *Gynecol. Oncol.* **1999**, *75*, 198–210. [CrossRef]
58. Vindevogel, E.; Baert, T.; Van Hoylandt, A.; Verbist, G.; Velde, G.V.; Garg, A.D.; Agostinis, P.; Vergote, I.; Coosemans, A.N. The Use of Toll-like Receptor 4 Agonist to Reshape the Immune Signature in Ovarian Cancer. *Anticancer Res.* **2016**, *36*, 5781–5792. [CrossRef]
59. Zhang, Y.-M.; Rock, C.O. Membrane lipid homeostasis in bacteria. *Nat. Rev. Genet.* **2008**, *6*, 222–233. [CrossRef]
60. Zheng, L.; Lin, Y.; Lu, S.; Zhang, J.; Bogdanov, M. Biogenesis, transport and remodeling of lysophospholipids in Gram-negative bacteria. *Biochim. Biophys. Acta (BBA) Mol. Cell Biol. Lipids* **2017**, *1862*, 1404–1413. [CrossRef]
61. Fan, L.; Zhang, W.; Yin, M.; Zhang, T.; Wu, X.; Zhang, H.; Sun, M.; Li, Z.; Hou, Y.; Zhou, X.; et al. Identification of metabolic biomarkers to diagnose epithelial ovarian cancer using a UPLC/QTOF/MS platform. *Acta Oncol.* **2012**, *51*, 473–479. [CrossRef] [PubMed]
62. Zhang, T.; Wu, X.; Ke, C.; Yin, M.; Li, Z.; Fan, L.; Zhang, W.; Zhang, H.; Zhao, F.; Zhou, X.; et al. Identification of Potential Biomarkers for Ovarian Cancer by Urinary Metabolomic Profiling. *J. Proteome Res.* **2013**, *12*, 505–512. [CrossRef] [PubMed]
63. Lee, Z.; Swaby, R.F.; Liang, Y.; Yu, S.; Liu, S.; Lu, K.H.; Bast, R.C.; Mills, G.B.; Fang, X. Lysophosphatidic Acid is a Major Regulator of Growth-Regulated Oncogene α in Ovarian Cancer. *Cancer Res* **2006**, *66*, 2740–2748. [CrossRef] [PubMed]
64. Xu, Y.; Fang, X.J.; Casey, G.; Mills, G.B. Lysophospholipids activate ovarian and breast cancer cells. *Biochem. J.* **1995**, *309 Pt 3*, 933–940. [CrossRef] [PubMed]
65. Estrella, V.C.; Eder, A.M.; Liu, S.; Pustilnik, T.B.; Tabassam, F.H.; Claret, F.X.; Gallick, G.E.; Mills, G.B.; Wiener, J.R. Lysophosphatidic acid induction of urokinase plasminogen activator secretion requires activation of the p38MAPK pathway. *Int. J. Oncol.* **2007**, *31*, 441–449. [CrossRef] [PubMed]
66. Jeong, K.J.; Park, S.Y.; Cho, K.H.; Sohn, J.S.; Lee, J.; Kim, Y.K.; Kang, J.; Park, C.G.; Han, J.W.; Lee, H.Y. The Rho/ROCK pathway for lysophosphatidic acid-induced proteolytic enzyme expression and ovarian cancer cell invasion. *Oncogene* **2012**, *31*, 4279–4289. [CrossRef]
67. Jeong, G.O.; Shin, S.H.; Seo, E.J.; Kwon, Y.W.; Heo, S.C.; Kim, K.-H.; Yoon, M.-S.; Suh, D.-S.; Kim, J.H. TAZ Mediates Lysophosphatidic Acid-Induced Migration and Proliferation of Epithelial Ovarian Cancer Cells. *Cell. Physiol. Biochem.* **2013**, *32*, 253–263. [CrossRef]
68. Pustilnik, T.B.; Estrella, V.; Wiener, J.R.; Mao, M.; Eder, A.; Watt, A.M.; Bast, R.; Mills, G.B. Lysophosphatidic acid induces urokinase secretion by ovarian cancer cells. *Clin. Cancer Res.* **1999**, *5*, 3704–3710.
69. Sengupta, S.; Xiao, Y.J.; Xu, Y. A novel laminin-induced LPA autocrine loop in the migration of ovarian cancer cells. *Faseb J.* **2003**, *17*, 1570–1572. [CrossRef]
70. Hurst, J.H.; Hooks, S.B. Lysophosphatidic Acid Stimulates Cell Growth by Different Mechanisms in SKOV-3 and Caov-3 Ovarian Cancer Cells: Distinct Roles for Gi- and Rho-Dependent Pathways. *Pharmacology* **2009**, *83*, 333–347. [CrossRef]
71. Wikoff, W.R.; Anfora, A.T.; Liu, J.; Schultz, P.G.; Lesley, S.A.; Peters, E.C.; Siuzdak, G. Metabolomics analysis reveals large effects of gut microflora on mammalian blood metabolites. *Proc. Natl. Acad. Sci. USA* **2009**, *106*, 3698–3703. [CrossRef]
72. Yokoyama, M.T.; Carlson, J.R. Microbial metabolites of tryptophan in the intestinal tract with special reference to skatole. *Am. J. Clin. Nutr.* **1979**, *32*, 173–178. [CrossRef]
73. Browne, C.A.; Clarke, G.; Dinan, T.G.; Cryan, J.F. An effective dietary method for chronic tryptophan depletion in two mouse strains illuminates a role for 5-HT in nesting behaviour. *Neuropharmacology* **2012**, *62*, 1903–1915. [CrossRef]

74. El Aidy, S.; Kunze, W.; Bienenstock, J.; Kleerebezem, M. The microbiota and the gut-brain axis: Insights from the temporal and spatial mucosal alterations during colonisation of the germfree mouse intestine. *Benef. Microbes* **2012**, *3*, 251–259. [CrossRef]
75. Mardinoglu, A.; Shoaie, S.; Bergentall, M.; Ghaffari, P.; Zhang, C.; Larsson, E.; Bäckhed, F.; Nielsen, J. The gut microbiota modulates host amino acid and glutathione metabolism in mice. *Mol. Syst. Biol.* **2015**, *11*, 834. [CrossRef]
76. Gao, J.; Xu, K.; Liu, H.; Liu, G.; Bai, M.; Peng, C.; Li, T.; Yin, Y. Impact of the gut microbiota on intestinal immunity mediated by tryptophan metabolism. *Front. Cell Infect Microbiol.* **2018**, *8*, 13. [CrossRef] [PubMed]
77. Zelante, T.; Iannitti, R.G.; Cunha, C.; De Luca, A.; Giovannini, G.; Pierraccini, G.; Zecchi, R.; D'Angelo, C.; Massi-Benedetti, C.; Fallarino, F.; et al. Tryptophan catabolites from microbiota engage aryl hydrocarbon receptor and balance mucosal reactivity via interleukin-22. *Immunity* **2013**, *39*, 372–385. [CrossRef] [PubMed]
78. Venkatesh, M.; Mukherjee, S.; Wang, H.; Li, H.; Sun, K.; Benechet, A.P.; Qiu, Z.; Maher, L.; Redinbo, M.R.; Phillips, R.S.; et al. Symbiotic Bacterial Metabolites Regulate Gastrointestinal Barrier Function via the Xenobiotic Sensor PXR and Toll-like Receptor 4. *Immunity* **2014**, *41*, 296–310. [CrossRef] [PubMed]
79. Lamas, B.; Richard, M.L.; Leducq, V.; Pham, H.-P.; Michel, M.-L.; Da Costa, G.; Bridonneau, C.; Jegou, S.; Hoffmann, T.W.; Natividad, J.M.; et al. CARD9 impacts colitis by altering gut microbiota metabolism of tryptophan into aryl hydrocarbon receptor ligands. *Nat. Med.* **2016**, *22*, 598–605. [CrossRef]
80. Kim, C.H. Immune regulation by microbiome metabolites. *Immunology* **2018**, *154*, 220–229. [CrossRef]
81. Shi, L.Z.; Faith, N.G.; Nakayama, Y.; Suresh, M.; Steinberg, H.; Czuprynski, C.J. The Aryl Hydrocarbon Receptor Is Required for Optimal Resistance to *Listeria monocytogenes* Infection in Mice. *J. Immunol.* **2007**, *179*, 6952–6962. [CrossRef]
82. Qiu, J.; Heller, J.J.; Guo, X.; Chen, Z.-M.E.; Fish, K.; Fu, Y.-X.; Zhou, L. The Aryl Hydrocarbon Receptor Regulates Gut Immunity through Modulation of Innate Lymphoid Cells. *Immunity* **2012**, *36*, 92–104. [CrossRef]
83. Zhang, L.; Nichols, R.; Patterson, A.D. The aryl hydrocarbon receptor as a moderator of host-microbiota communication. *Curr. Opin. Toxicol.* **2017**, *2*, 30–35. [CrossRef] [PubMed]
84. Plewa, S.; Horała, A.; Dereziński, P.; Klupczynska, A.; Nowak-Markwitz, E.; Matysiak, J.; Kokot, Z.J. Usefulness of Amino Acid Profiling in Ovarian Cancer Screening with Special Emphasis on Their Role in Cancerogenesis. *Int. J. Mol. Sci.* **2017**, *18*, 2727. [CrossRef] [PubMed]
85. Hilvo, M.; de Santiago, I.; Gopalacharyulu, P.; Schmitt, W.D.; Budczies, J.; Kuhberg, M.; Dietel, M.; Aittokallio, T.; Markowetz, F.; Denkert, C.; et al. Accumulated Metabolites of Hydroxybutyric Acid Serve as Diagnostic and Prognostic Biomarkers of Ovarian High-Grade Serous Carcinomas. *Cancer Res.* **2016**, *76*, 796–804. [CrossRef] [PubMed]
86. Zhou, M.; Guan, W.; Walker, L.D.; Mezencev, R.; Benigno, B.B.; Gray, A.; Fernández, F.M.; McDonald, J.F. Rapid Mass Spectrometric Metabolic Profiling of Blood Sera Detects Ovarian Cancer with High Accuracy. *Cancer Epidemiol. Biomark. Prev.* **2010**, *19*, 2262–2271. [CrossRef]
87. Zhang, T.; Wu, X.; Yin, M.; Fan, L.; Zhang, H.; Zhao, F.; Zhang, W.; Ke, C.; Zhang, G.; Hou, Y.; et al. Discrimination between malignant and benign ovarian tumors by plasma metabolomic profiling using ultra performance liquid chromatography/mass spectrometry. *Clin. Chim. Acta* **2012**, *413*, 861–868. [CrossRef]
88. Ke, C.; Hou, Y.; Zhang, H.; Fan, L.; Ge, T.; Guo, B.; Zhang, F.; Yang, K.; Wang, J.; Lou, G.; et al. Large-scale profiling of metabolic dysregulation in ovarian cancer. *Int. J. Cancer* **2014**, *136*, 516–526. [CrossRef]
89. Lamb, R.; Ozsvari, B.; Lisanti, C.L.; Tanowitz, H.B.; Howell, A.; Martinez-Outschoorn, U.E.; Sotgia, F.; Lisanti, M.P. Antibiotics that target mitochondria effectively eradicate cancer stem cells, across multiple tumor types: Treating cancer like an infectious disease. *Oncotarget* **2015**, *6*, 4569–4584. [CrossRef]
90. Ataie-Kachoie, P.; Badar, S.; Morris, D.L.; Pourgholami, M.H. Minocycline targets the NF-κB Nexus through suppression of TGF-β1-TAK1-IκB signaling in ovarian cancer. *Mol. Cancer Res.* **2013**, *11*, 1279–1291. [CrossRef]
91. Ataie-Kachoie, P.; Morris, D.L.; Pourgholami, M.H. Minocycline Suppresses Interleukine-6, Its Receptor System and Signaling Pathways and Impairs Migration, Invasion and Adhesion Capacity of Ovarian Cancer Cells: In Vitro and In Vivo Studies. *PLoS ONE* **2013**, *8*, e60817. [CrossRef] [PubMed]
92. Ataie-Kachoie, P.; Pourgholami, M.H.; Bahrami-B, F.; Badar, S.; Morris, D.L. Minocycline attenuates hypoxia-inducible factor-1α expression correlated with modulation of p53 and AKT/mTOR/p70S6K/4E-BP1 pathway in ovarian cancer: In vitro and in vivo studies. *Am. J. Cancer Res.* **2015**, *5*, 575–588. [PubMed]
93. Pourgholami, M.H.; Ataie-Kachoie, P.; Badar, S.; Morris, D.L. Minocycline inhibits malignant ascites of ovarian cancer through targeting multiple signaling pathways. *Gynecol. Oncol.* **2013**, *129*, 113–119. [CrossRef] [PubMed]
94. Kloskowski, T.; Olkowska, J.; Nazlica, A.; Drewa, T. The influence of ciprofloxacin on hamster ovarian cancer cell line CHO AA8. *Acta Pol. Pharm.-Drug Res.* **2010**, *67*, 345–349.
95. Parajuli, B.; Lee, H.-G.; Kwon, S.-H.; Cha, S.-D.; Shin, S.-J.; Lee, G.-H.; Bae, I.; Cho, C.-H. Salinomycin inhibits Akt/NF-κB and induces apoptosis in cisplatin resistant ovarian cancer cells. *Cancer Epidemiol.* **2013**, *37*, 512–517. [CrossRef]
96. Parajuli, B.; Shin, S.-J.; Kwon, S.-H.; Cha, S.-D.; Chung, R.; Park, W.-J.; Lee, H.-G.; Cho, C.-H. Salinomycin induces apoptosis via death receptor-5 up-regulation in cisplatin-resistant ovarian cancer cells. *Anticancer Res.* **2013**, *33*, 1457–1462.
97. Chung, H.; Kim, Y.-H.; Kwon, M.; Shin, S.-J.; Kwon, S.-H.; Cha, S.-D.; Cho, C.-H. The effect of salinomycin on ovarian cancer stem-like cells. *Obstet. Gynecol. Sci.* **2016**, *59*, 261–268. [CrossRef]
98. Kaplan, F.; Teksen, F. Apoptotic effects of salinomycin on human ovarian cancer cell line (OVCAR-3). *Tumor Biol.* **2015**, *37*, 3897–3903. [CrossRef]

99. Li, R.; Dong, T.; Hu, C.; Lu, J.; Dai, J.; Liu, P. Salinomycin repressed the epithelial–mesenchymal transition of epithelial ovarian cancer cells via downregulating Wnt/β-catenin pathway. *OncoTargets Ther.* **2017**, *10*, 1317–1325. [CrossRef]
100. Lee, H.-G.; Shin, S.-J.; Chung, H.-W.; Kwon, S.-H.; Cha, S.-D.; Lee, J.-E.; Cho, C.-H. Salinomycin reduces stemness and induces apoptosis on human ovarian cancer stem cell. *J. Gynecol. Oncol.* **2017**, *28*, e14. [CrossRef]
101. Chambers, L.M.; Rhoades, E.E.; Bharti, R.; Braley, C.; Tewari, S.; Trestan, L.; Alali, Z.; Bayik, D.; Lathia, J.; Sangwan, N.; et al. Disruption of the gut microbiota attenuates epithelial ovarian cancer sensitivity to cisplatin therapy. *bioRxiv* **2020**, *82*, 4654–4669.
102. Huang, H.-C.; Liu, J.; Baglo, Y.; Rizvi, I.; Anbil, S.; Pigula, M.; Hasan, T. Mechanism-informed Repurposing of Minocycline Overcomes Resistance to Topoisomerase Inhibition for Peritoneal Carcinomatosis. *Mol. Cancer Ther.* **2018**, *17*, 508–520. [CrossRef] [PubMed]
103. Xu, S.; Liu, Z.; Lv, M.; Chen, Y.; Liu, Y. Intestinal dysbiosis promotes epithelial-mesenchymal transition by activating tumor-associated macrophages in ovarian cancer. *Pathog. Dis.* **2019**, *77*. [CrossRef] [PubMed]
104. Walboomers, J.M.; Jacobs, M.V.; Manos, M.M.; Bosch, F.X.; Kummer, J.A.; Shah, K.V.; Snijders, P.J.; Peto, J.; Meijer, C.J.; Muñoz, N. Human papillomavirus is a necessary cause of invasive cervical cancer worldwide. *J Pathol.* **1999**, *189*, 12–19. [CrossRef]
105. Mitra, A.; MacIntyre, D.A.; Lee, Y.S.; Smith, A.; Marchesi, J.R.; Lehne, B.; Bhatia, R.; Lyons, D.; Paraskevaidis, E.; Li, J.V.; et al. Cervical intraepithelial neoplasia disease progression is associated with increased vaginal microbiome diversity. *Sci. Rep.* **2015**, *5*, 1–11. [CrossRef] [PubMed]
106. Gillet, E.; Meys, J.F.; Verstraelen, H.; Bosire, C.; De Sutter, P.; Temmerman, M.; Broeck, D.V. Bacterial vaginosis is associated with uterine cervical human papillomavirus infection: A meta-analysis. *BMC Infect. Dis.* **2011**, *11*, 10. [CrossRef]
107. Guo, Y.-L.; You, K.; Qiao, J.; Zhao, Y.-m.; Geng, L. Bacterial vaginosis is conducive to the persistence of HPV infection. *Int. J. STD AIDS* **2012**, *23*, 581–584. [CrossRef]
108. Norenhag, J.; Du, J.; Olovsson, M.; Verstraelen, H.; Engstrand, L.; Brusselaers, N. The vaginal microbiota, human papillomavirus and cervical dysplasia: A systematic review and network meta-analysis. *BJOG Int. J. Obstet. Gynaecol.* **2020**, *127*, 171–180. [CrossRef]
109. Borella, F.; Carosso, A.R.; Cosma, S.; Preti, M.; Collemi, G.; Cassoni, P.; Bertero, L.; Benedetto, C. Gut Microbiota and Gynecological Cancers: A Summary of Pathogenetic Mechanisms and Future Directions. *ACS Infect. Dis.* **2021**, *7*, 987–1009. [CrossRef]
110. Di Paola, M.; Sani, C.; Clemente, A.M.; Iossa, A.; Perissi, E.; Castronovo, G.; Tanturli, M.; Rivero, D.; Cozzolino, F.; Cavalieri, D.; et al. Characterization of cervico-vaginal microbiota in women developing persistent high-risk Human Papillomavirus infection. *Sci. Rep.* **2017**, *7*, 10200. [CrossRef]
111. Round, J.L.; Mazmanian, S.K. The gut microbiota shapes intestinal immune responses during health and disease. *Nat. Rev. Immunol.* **2009**, *9*, 313–323. [CrossRef] [PubMed]
112. Torcia, M.G. Interplay among Vaginal Microbiome, Immune Response and Sexually Transmitted Viral Infections. *Int. J. Mol. Sci.* **2019**, *20*, 266. [CrossRef] [PubMed]
113. Wiik, J.; Sengpiel, V.; Kyrgiou, M.; Nilsson, S.; Mitra, A.; Tanbo, T.; Jonassen, C.M.; Tannæs, T.M.; Sjøborg, K. Cervical microbiota in women with cervical intra-epithelial neoplasia, prior to and after local excisional treatment, a Norwegian cohort study. *BMC Women's Heal.* **2019**, *19*, 1–9. [CrossRef] [PubMed]
114. Klein, C.; Gonzalez, D.; Samwel, K.; Kahesa, C.; Mwaiselage, J.; Aluthge, N.; Fernando, S.; West, J.T.; Wood, C.; Angeletti, P.C. Relationship between the Cervical Microbiome, HIV Status, and Precancerous Lesions. *mBio* **2019**, *10*, e02785-18. [CrossRef]
115. Verteramo, R.; Pierangeli, A.; Mancini, E.; Calzolari, E.; Bucci, M.; Osborn, J.; Degener, R.; Chiarini, F.; Antonelli, G.; Degener, A.M. Human Papillomaviruses and genital co-infections in gynaecological outpatients. *BMC Infect. Dis.* **2009**, *9*, 16. [CrossRef]
116. Samoff, E.; Koumans, E.H.; Markowitz, L.E.; Maya, S.; Sawyer, M.K.; Swan, D.; Papp, J.R.; Black, C.M.; Unger, E.R. Association of Chlamydia trachomatis with persistence of high-risk types of human Papillomavirus in a cohort of female adolescents. *Am. J. Epidemiol.* **2005**, *162*, 668. [CrossRef]
117. Paavonen, J. *Chlamydia trachomatis* infections of the female genital tract: State of the art. *Ann. Med.* **2011**, *44*, 18–28. [CrossRef]
118. Audirac-Chalifour, A.; Torres-Poveda, K.; Bahena-Román, M.; Téllez-Sosa, J.; Martínez-Barnetche, J.; Cortina-Ceballos, B.; López-Estrada, G.; Delgado-Romero, K.; Burguete-García, A.I.; Cantú, D.; et al. Cervical Microbiome and Cytokine Profile at Various Stages of Cervical Cancer: A Pilot Study. *PLoS ONE* **2016**, *11*, e0153274. [CrossRef]
119. Routy, B.; Le Chatelier, E.; Derosa, L.; Duong, C.P.M.; Alou, M.T.; Daillère, R.; Fluckiger, A.; Messaoudene, M.; Rauber, C.; Roberti, M.P.; et al. Gut microbiome influences efficacy of PD-1-based immunotherapy against epithelial tumors. *Science* **2018**, *359*, 91–97. [CrossRef]
120. Santoni, M.; Piva, F.; Conti, A.; Santoni, A.; Cimadamore, A.; Scarpelli, M.; Battelli, N.; Montironi, R. Re: Gut Microbiome Influences Efficacy of PD-1-based Immunotherapy Against Epithelial Tumors. *Eur. Urol.* **2018**, *74*, 521–522. [CrossRef]
121. Sivan, A.; Corrales, L.; Hubert, N.; Williams, J.B.; Aquino-Michaels, K.; Earley, Z.M.; Benyamin, F.W.; Lei, Y.M.; Jabri, B.; Alegre, M.-L.; et al. Commensal Bifidobacterium promotes antitumor immunity and facilitates anti-PD-L1 efficacy. *Science* **2015**, *350*, 1084–1089. [CrossRef] [PubMed]
122. Kim, S.-J.; Kang, C.-H.; Kim, G.-H.; Cho, H. Anti-Tumor Effects of Heat-Killed L. reuteri MG5346 and L. casei MG4584 against Human Colorectal Carcinoma through Caspase-9-Dependent Apoptosis in Xenograft Model. *Microorganisms* **2022**, *10*, 533. [CrossRef] [PubMed]
123. Chilakapati, S.R.; Ricciuti, J.; Zsiros, E. Microbiome and cancer immunotherapy. *Curr. Opin. Biotechnol.* **2020**, *65*, 114–117. [CrossRef] [PubMed]

124. Gopalakrishnan, V.; Spencer, C.N.; Nezi, L.; Reuben, A.; Andrews, M.C.; Karpinets, T.V.; Prieto, P.A.; Vicente, D.; Hoffman, K.; Wei, S.C.; et al. Gut microbiome modulates response to anti–PD-1 immunotherapy in melanoma patients. *Science* **2018**, *359*, 97–103. [CrossRef] [PubMed]
125. Alexander, J.L.; Wilson, I.D.; Teare, J.; Marchesi, J.R.; Nicholson, J.K.; Kinross, J.M. Gut microbiota modulation of chemotherapy efficacy and toxicity. *Nat. Rev. Gastroenterol. Hepatol.* **2017**, *14*, 356–365. [CrossRef] [PubMed]
126. Wilkinson, E.M.; Ilhan, Z.E.; Herbst-Kralovetz, M.M. Microbiota–drug interactions: Impact on metabolism and efficacy of therapeutics. *Maturitas* **2018**, *112*, 53–63. [CrossRef]
127. Weiman, S. *Harnessing the Power of Microbes as Therapeutics: Bugs as Drugs: Report on an American Academy of Microbiology Colloquium Held in San Diego, CA, in April 2014*; Fox, J., Ed.; American Society for Microbiology: Washington, DC, USA, 2015.
128. Carvalho, R.; Vaz, A.; Pereira, F.L.; Dorella, F.; Aguiar, E.; Chatel, J.-M.; Bermudez, L.; Langella, P.; Fernandes, G.; Figueiredo, H.; et al. Gut microbiome modulation during treatment of mucositis with the dairy bacterium Lactococcus lactis and recombinant strain secreting human antimicrobial PAP. *Sci. Rep.* **2018**, *8*, 15072. [CrossRef] [PubMed]
129. Cui, M.; Xiao, H.; Li, Y.; Zhou, L.; Zhao, S.; Luo, D.; Zheng, Q.; Dong, J.; Zhao, Y.; Zhang, X.; et al. Faecal microbiota transplantation protects against radiation-induced toxicity. *EMBO Mol. Med.* **2017**, *9*, 448–461. [CrossRef]
130. Biancheri, P.; Divekar, D.; Watson, A.J. Could Fecal Transplantation Become Part of PD-1-Based Immunotherapy, Due to Effects of the Intestinal Microbiome? *Gastroenterology* **2018**, *154*, 1845–1847. [CrossRef]
131. Hemmerling, A.; Harrison, W.; Schroeder, A.; Park, J.; Korn, A.; Shiboski, S.; Foster-Rosales, A.; Cohen, C.R. Phase 2a Study Assessing Colonization Efficiency, Safety, and Acceptability of Lactobacillus crispatus CTV-05 in Women With Bacterial Vaginosis. *Sex. Transm. Dis.* **2010**, *37*, 745–750. [CrossRef]
132. Stapleton, A.E.; Au-Yeung, M.; Hooton, T.M.; Fredricks, D.N.; Roberts, P.L.; Czaja, C.A.; Yarova-Yarovaya, Y.; Fiedler, T.; Cox, M.; Stamm, W.E. Randomized, Placebo-Controlled Phase 2 Trial of a Lactobacillus crispatus Probiotic Given Intravaginally for Prevention of Recurrent Urinary Tract Infection. *Clin. Infect. Dis.* **2011**, *52*, 1212–1217. [CrossRef] [PubMed]
133. Qingqing, B.; Jie, Z.; Songben, Q.; Juan, C.; Lei, Z.; Mu, X. Cervicovaginal microbiota dysbiosis correlates with HPV persistent infection. *Microb. Pathog.* **2020**, *152*, 104617. [CrossRef] [PubMed]
134. Zeng, M.; Li, X.; Jiao, X.; Cai, X.; Yao, F.; Xu, S.; Huang, X.; Zhang, Q.; Chen, J. Roles of vaginal flora in human papillomavirus infection, virus persistence and clearance. *Front. Cell. Infect. Microbiol.* **2023**, *12*, 104617. [CrossRef] [PubMed]
135. Palma, E.; Recine, N.; Domenici, L.; Giorgini, M.; Pierangeli, A.; Panici, P.B. Long-term Lactobacillus rhamnosus BMX 54 application to restore a balanced vaginal ecosystem: A promising solution against HPV-infection. *BMC Infect. Dis.* **2018**, *18*, 13. [CrossRef]
136. Tsementzi, D.; Pena-Gonzalez, A.; Bai, J.; Hu, Y.J.; Patel, P.; Shelton, J.; Dolan, M.; Arluck, J.; Khanna, N.; Conrad, L.; et al. Comparison of vaginal microbiota in gynecologic cancer patients pre- and post-radiation therapy and healthy women. *Cancer Med.* **2020**, *9*, 3714–3724. [CrossRef]
137. Yuan, M.; Li, D.; Zhang, Z.; Sun, H.; An, M.; Wang, G. Endometriosis induces gut microbiota alterations in mice. *Hum Reprod Oxf Engl.* **2018**, *33*, 607–616. [CrossRef]
138. Jiang, I.; Yong, P.J.; Allaire, C.; Bedaiwy, M.A. Intricate Connections between the Microbiota and Endometriosis. *Int. J. Mol. Sci.* **2021**, *22*, 5644. [CrossRef]

Disclaimer/Publisher's Note: The statements, opinions and data contained in all publications are solely those of the individual author(s) and contributor(s) and not of MDPI and/or the editor(s). MDPI and/or the editor(s) disclaim responsibility for any injury to people or property resulting from any ideas, methods, instructions or products referred to in the content.

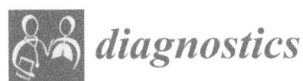

Article

HPV-Induced Anal and Peri-Anal Neoplasia, a Surgeon's Experience: 5-Year Case Series

Christoforos Kosmidis [1], Christina Sevva [1,*], Vasiliki Magra [1], Nikolaos Varsamis [2], Charilaos Koulouris [1], Ioannis Charalampous [1], Konstantinos Papadopoulos [1], Panagiota Roulia [1], Marios Dagher [1], Vasiliki Theodorou [3], Chrysi Maria Mystakidou [3] and Isaak Kesisoglou [1]

[1] 3rd Surgical Department, University General Hospital of Thessaloniki "AHEPA", School of Medicine, Faculty of Health Sciences, Aristotle University of Thessaloniki, 1st St. Kiriakidi Street, 54621 Thessaloniki, Greece
[2] European Interbalkan Medical Center, 10 Asklipiou Street, 55535 Pylaia, Greece
[3] Medical School, Faculty of Health Sciences, Aristotle University of Thessaloniki, 54124 Thessaloniki, Greece
* Correspondence: christina.sevva@gmail.com

Abstract: *Purpose*: One of the most known sexually transmitted diseases is Condylomata acuminata (CA), a skin lesion occurring due to infection from Human Papilloma Virus (HPV). CA has a typical appearance of raised, skin-colored papules ranging in size from 1 mm to 5 mm. These lesions often form cauliflower-like plaques. Depending on the involved HPV-subtype (either high-risk or low-risk) and its malignant potential, these lesions are likely to lead to malignant transformation when specific HPV subtypes and other risk factors are present. Therefore, high clinical suspicion is required when examining the anal and perianal area. *Methods*: In this article, the authors aim to present the results of a five-year case series (2016–2021) of anal and perianal cases of CA. *Results*: A total of 35 patients were included in this study. Patients were categorized based on specific criteria, which included gender, sex preferences, and human immunodeficiency virus infection. All patients underwent proctoscopy and excision biopsies were obtained. Based on dysplasia grade patients were further categorized. The group of patients where high-dysplasia squamous cell carcinoma was present was initially treated with chemoradiotherapy. Abdominoperineal resection was necessary in five cases after local recurrence. *Conclusions*: CA remains a serious condition where several treatment options are available if detected early. Delay in diagnosis can lead to malignant transformation, often leaving abdominoperineal resection as the only option. Vaccination against HPV poses a key role in eliminating the transmission of the virus, and thus the prevalence of CA.

Keywords: condylomata acuminata; HPV; abdominoperineal resection; vaccination

1. Introduction

Condylomata acuminata (CA), otherwise known as anogenital warts, are caused by human papilloma virus (HPV) infection. HPV is one of the commonest sexually transmitted diseases worldwide, with 9–13% of the world population affected [1,2], commonly between 20 and 39 years old [1].

HPV is a non-enveloped, double-stranded DNA virus from the papilloma virus family that infects the nucleus of differentiated squamous cells [1,3]. It can remain in a latent state, with an incubation period from one month to two years after infection [1]. More than 200 [3] subtypes have been described, which are subdivided into high-risk (HR-HPV) and low-risk types (LR-HPV) based on their oncogenic potential [4]. More than 40 types are known to affect the anogenital area [1]. Low-risk types 6 and 11 are responsible for over 90% of condylomata acuminata [4]. High-risk types 16 and 18 have been solidly linked to cervical, anal, and oral malignancy [4]. HPV infection appears to be the cause for most anal cancers and virtually all cases of cervical cancer [5]. Due to its structure, the viral DNA integrates into the host human genome causing malignant transformation and

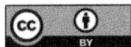

eventually evolving to cancer. Evolution to cancer occurs mostly through actions affecting two major paths: alterations in cell cycle regulation and telomeres combined with blockage in apoptosis. These interventions cause DNA instability, leading eventually to genomic damage, and together with the disabled tumor suppressor paths, mostly protein p53, result in the progression to malignancies [6,7].

The HPV genome consists of a transcribed region which encodes six early proteins, namely E1, E2, E4, E5, E6, and E7. Some of these HPV proteins are strongly type-specific and they can be detected in certain neoplastic lesions. Especially in the HR-HPV subtypes increased levels of E5, E6, and E7 oncoproteins seem to affect and activate multiple signaling pathways and thus stimulate proliferation of infected cells. Although life-cycle organization between HR- and LR-HPV subtypes is similar, the main difference lies in the strongly different ability of each group's oncoproteins (mostly E6 and E7) to control cell cycle entry in the basal/parabasal cell layers [8,9].

HPV invades the cells of the epidermal basal layer through microabrasions [3]. Transmission occurs via human-to-human contact, smear infection, or vertically [4]. Several types of HPV exist which show a different biological behavior. Based on this behavior, the HPV subtypes are further categorized into low-risk and high-risk types according to their malignant potential. Low-risk types (also known as non-oncogenic types) include HPV 6, 11, 40, 42, 43, 44, 54, 61, 70, 72, 81, and CP6108 and are mainly responsible for causing anogenital warts, low-grade changes in cells of the cervix and recurrent respiratory papillomatosis [6,10]. The oncogenic high-risk HPV types include HPV 16, 18, 31, 33, 35, 39, 45, 51, 52, 56, 58, 59, 66, 68, 73, and 82. HPV 16 and 18 seem to have the higher malignant potential as they are linked with high-grade dysplasia and invasive carcinoma of the cervix and the anus in both men and women [6,11].

High-risk HPV subtypes are responsible for certain types of cancer of the cervix (cervical intraepithelial neoplasia (CIN)), anus, penis, vagina, vulva, oropharynx and even esophageal adenocarcinoma (EAC). Subtypes HPV-16 and HPV-18 are held responsible for the majority of cervical cancers and almost 95% of HPV-positive oropharyngeal cancers (OPCs). Other types of high-risk HPV related neoplasia are the vulvar high-grade squamous intraepithelial lesions (vH-SIL) which can progress to invasive vulvar cancer. From the low-risk HPV subtypes, some persistent ones, such as HPV-6 and HPV-11, cause recurrent conditions and mostly involve anogenital warts, respiratory papillomatosis, and vulvar low-grade squamous intraepithelial lesions (vL-SIL), which are considered to represent a benign condition [12,13].

Risk factors for infection include early-onset sexual contact, multiple sexual partners, high-risk sexual practices, concomitant infection with other sexually transmitted diseases (HIV, chlamydia, gonorrhea, HBV), and poor hygiene [4]. Regular use of condoms can protect against HPV infection but cannot fully prevent it. HPV vaccination prior to first sexual contact prevents infection with the subtypes contained in the vaccine. Available vaccines are the 9-valent for types 6, 11, 16, 18, 31, 33, 45, 52, 58 (Gardasil®9), the quadrivalent vaccine for types 6, 11, 16, and 18 (Gardasil®), and the bivalent vaccine for the high-risk types 16 and 18 (Cervarix®). In Greece, HPV vaccination is offered to girls 11–18 years old and boys and girls 11–26 with risk factors (HIV infection, transplant patients, history of malignancy, autoimmune disease, and immunocompromised patients) [14].

HPV contains an oncogene that triggers cell proliferation using the three major viral oncoproteins mentioned above (E5, E6, E7) [6]. As the number of infected cells increases, epidermal layers thicken, leading to the macroscopic appearance of condylomata acuminata [1]. CA are typically diagnosed clinically due to their characteristic appearance. They are raised, skin-coloured papules ranging in size from 1 mm to 5 mm. These can coalesce, forming cauliflower-like plaques. CA can be flat or pedunculated lesions (Figure 1). In rare cases, they can form giant lesions, taking up the entire anogenital region. In such cases, Buschke-Lowenstein tumors or Giant Condylomata Acuminata caused by HPV infection should be considered. Bushke-Lowenstein tumor is categorized by some authors as a rare form of highly differentiated squamous cell carcinoma (SCC), although a globally accepted definition is not available in the literature [15,16] (Figure 2). Assessment of anal and perianal lesions is not complete without proctoscopy and in some cases sigmoidoscopy in order to identify lesions in the anal canal. Regular follow-up should follow initial diagnosis and treatment as there is a 2–4% risk of malignant transformation.

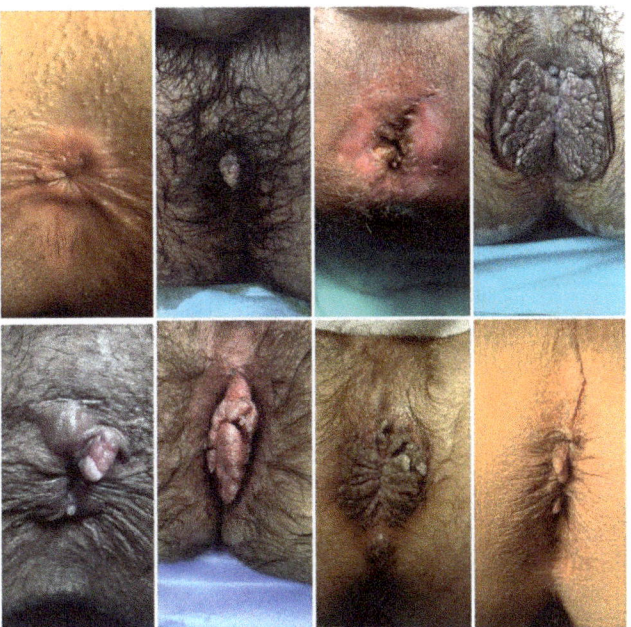

Figure 1. Different typical clinical presentation of CA as single papules or cauliflower-like plaques.

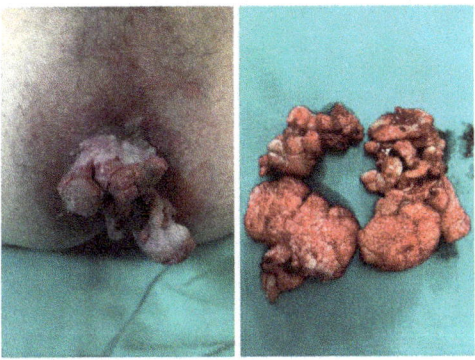

Figure 2. Clinical presentation of Giant CA (Bushke-Lowenstein tumor) and image of the specimen after excision.

Herein we present a 5-year case series (2016–2021) of anal and perianal CA.

2. Materials and Methods

The patients selected had surgical resection of anal and perianal warts between 1/1/2016 and 1/1/2021 (60 months) in the 3rd Surgical Department of University General Hospital of Thessaloniki AHEPA, by a single surgical team. Patient data were collected using the histopathological reports of the specimens resected, which were acquired from the Histopathology Laboratory of Aristotle University of Thessaloniki, along with the patient records from the 3rd Surgical Department's archive. Inclusion criteria included excision of anal and perianal lesions and exclusion criteria included final histopathological results of CA with high grade, mild-moderate dysplasia, and SCC.

3. Results

A total of 35 patients were included in this study. The patient cohort consisted mostly of men: 32 patients were male (91.4%) and three were female (8.6%), with an average age of 39.9 years. The patients were between the age of 17 and 73 years. Moreover, 13 of the male patients (37.1%) reported to have sex with men (MSM) (Figure 3 and Table 1. In addition, 15 patients were HIV positive (42.8%) (Figure 4 and Table 1). All HIV patients had CD4 levels in the normal range. None of the patients were immunized against HPV.

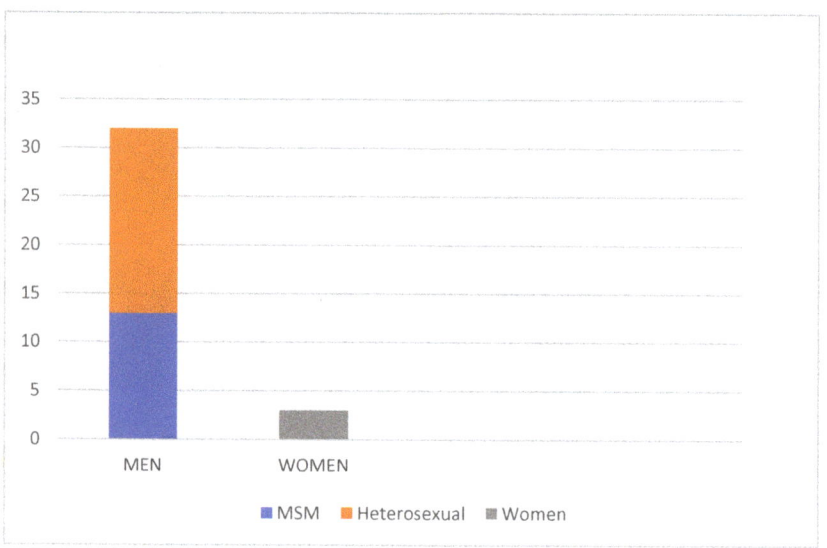

Figure 3. Distribution of the patients in our study based on sex. The vast majority being male (91.4%), 37% of which were MSM.

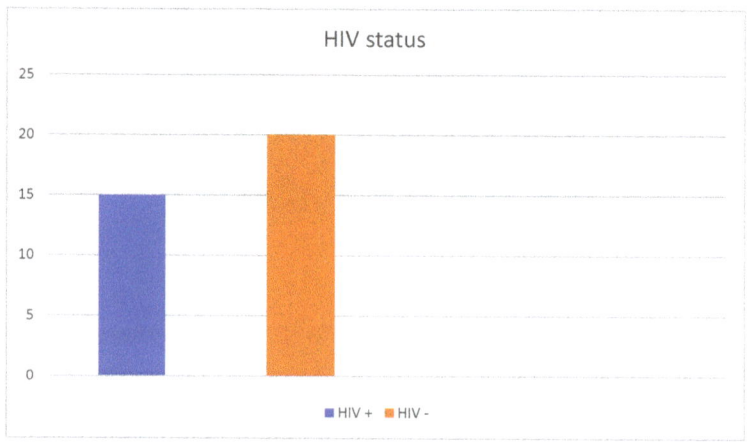

Figure 4. Prevalence of HIV in our patient cohort. Nearly half (42.8%) of the patients were HIV positive.

Table 1. Distribution of patients based on sex, sexual preferences and presence of HIV infection.

	Male (n = 32)	Female (n = 3)	Total (n = 35)
MSM	13	0	13
HIV (+)	15	0	15

All patients had proctoscopy under general anesthesia and excision biopsy of all suspicious perianal and anal lesions (Figure 5). Excision was performed using energy sources, specifically diathermy and radiofrequency-driven bipolar electrosurgical devices. All patients were administered topical agents, imiquimod or sinecatechins, post-operatively. All patients were followed up or remain subject to regular follow ups according to international guidelines for five years. Further, 16 patients required a second procedure to remove condylomata after relapse (45.7%) within this five-year follow up time period. All women treated were sent for a gynecology consult prior to excision biopsy and underwent a colposcopy and Pap smear test in order to rule out the presence of cervical intraepithelial neoplasia (CIN).

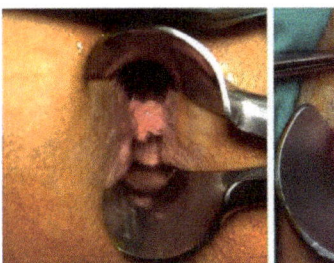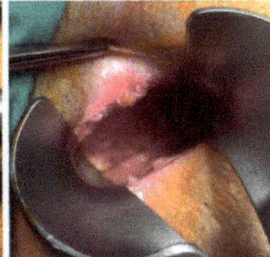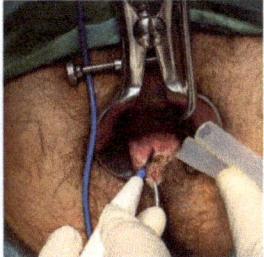

Figure 5. Lesions of CA revealed during proctoscopy using Eisenhammer Rectal Speculum.

Histopathology reports illustrate 16 patients with condylomata acuminata without dysplastic or neoplastic features (45.7%). Five patients had mid- to high grade dysplasia (14.3%); four patients had high grade dysplasia (11.4%); 10 patients (28.6%) were found to have invasive squamous cell carcinoma (SCC) in their histopathology results; two patients had Buschke-Lowenstein tumors (5.7%) (Figure 6 and Table 2. Interestingly enough, out of the 15 HIV (+) patients, only five appeared to have malignant lesions at the histopathological examination. However, not all of these malignant lesions showed a recurrent pattern in immunosuppressed patients. Four out of five patients that needed to undergo abdominoperineal resection appeared to be HIV (+). From the HIV (+) patients, five patients developed SCC, four patients showed some grade of dysplasia, and six patients developed no malignancies. Both the number of patients included and the number of immunosuppressed patients due to HIV infection are considered to be limited. Therefore, a safe correlation between HIV status and the occurrence of malignancy cannot be pointed out at this point. Patients with invasive SCC were initially treated with chemoradiotherapy, five (50%) of which required abdominoperineal resection after local recurrence. Three of the patients who underwent abdominoperineal resection remain disease free five years post-operatively, while the other two died in one and 3.5 years post-operatively, respectively (Figure 7 and Table 2).

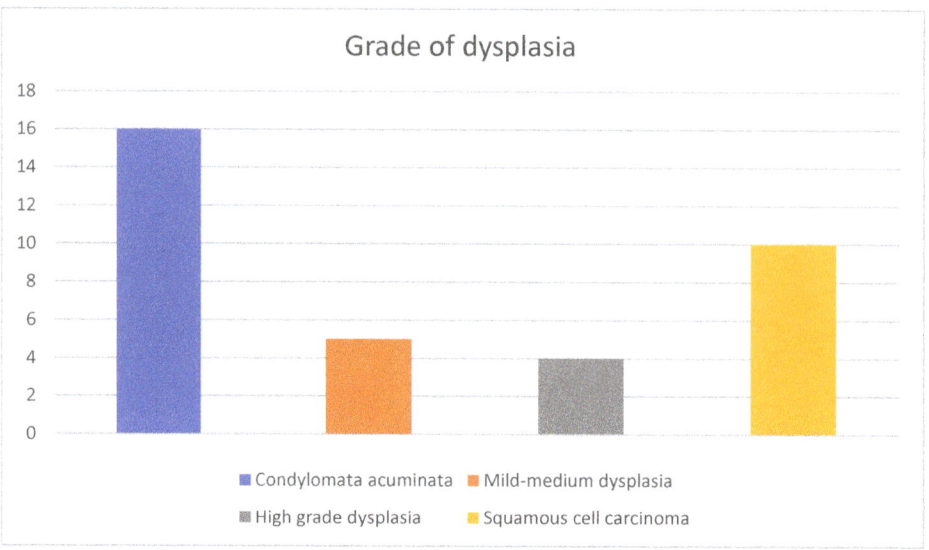

Figure 6. Grades of dysplasia in the histopathology results of the cohort, ranging from CA without dysplastic/neoplastic features to invasive SCC. A total of 19 patients (54.7%) had dysplastic and malignant features in their samples ranging from mild (5 patients) and high (4 patients) grade dysplasia to confirmed SCC (10 patients), illustrating the prevalence of malignant transformation in the context of CA and the importance of follow up.

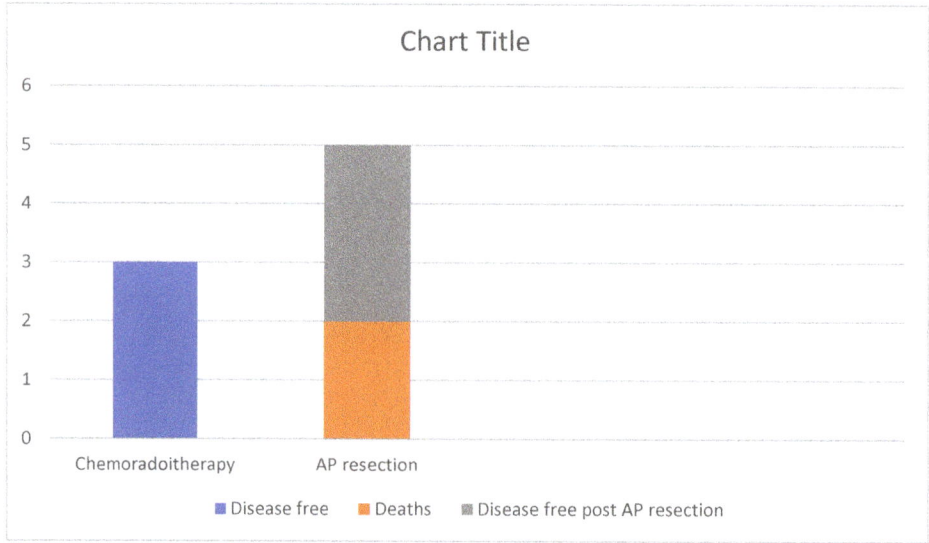

Figure 7. Outcomes of the patients with invasive SCC. 50% remain disease free after chemoradiotherapy alone, while of the 50% that required AP resection after relapse 60% remain disease free at 5 years post-operatively and 40% died.

Table 2. Outcomes of patients of the study.

	No Dysplasia (n = 16)	Mild Dysplasia (n = 5)	High Grade Dysplasia (n = 4)	SCC (n = 10)	Total (n = 35)
Chemoradiotherapy	-			10	10
Relapse + Abdominoperineal resection	-	-	-	5	5
Disease free	16	5	4	8	33
Deaths	-	-	-	2	2

The remaining 25 patients whose histopathology results showed no presence of confirmed malignancy did not receive any further treatment. Excision of the lesions was considered enough. These patients continue to have annual follow ups with proctoscopy and remain disease-free.

4. Discussion

Anal and perianal condylomata acuminata represent a controversial subject, largely due to limited clinical trials and high-level evidence, especially in terms of screening and prevention. There are currently no official guidelines regarding large scale vaccination for males and screening for anal SCC or HSIL (high grade squamous intraepithelial lesions). Although gender distribution appears to be roughly equal in the literature, the vast majority of the patients in this cohort were male (91.4%). This could be due to a number of factors. Nowadays, most women have regular screening for cervical cancer and consult their gynecologist frequently, who may manage a significant number of perianal warts. This department has a close cooperation with the HIV Medicine Unit of Aristotle University of Thessaloniki, which could account for the increased male predominance as well as the high percentage of HIV positive patients in this cohort.

Another significant observation to note is the large percentage of HSIL and invasive SCC. Interestingly, only a 2–4% rate of malignant transformation is reported in the literature, whereas we found 28.6% of our patient cohort had invasive SCC and nine patients (25.7%) had mid- to high grade dysplasia. HIV infection could, of course, contribute to the notably high percentage of dysplasia and invasive SCC, as it has been shown to be a risk factor for malignant transformation of CA [17–19]. There are currently no national standards for screening for HSIL or anal cancer in any country and insufficient evidence to support it from current literature [20–22]. However, recommendations for screening HIV positive patients with annual digital rectal examination, anoscopy, and/or anal Papanicolaou tests have been published by several organizations specializing in sexually transmitted infections (STIs) and colorectal diseases [20]. Clinical guidelines in regard to screening are expected to become more specific once the Anal Cancer HSIL (High-Grade Squamous Intraepithelial Lesions) Outcomes Research (ANCHOR) study is published [19,23,24]. The study started as a randomized clinical trial, which has been halted due to the therapy's high success rates. It is a large phase 3 study awaiting publication.

Patient information and prevention remains poor. Current HPV vaccination guidelines in Greece include girls from 11 to 18 years old as well as boys and girls from 11 to 26 years old in high-risk groups (patients with autoimmune diseases, on immunosuppressant treatment, HIV positive, patients with malignancy and transplant patients) [10,23]. The mean age of our cohort (39.9 years) is higher than mean age of infection, but it remains striking that none of the patients were vaccinated, especially as the youngest was 17 years old. This reflects the level of information and possibly the lack of availability of the vaccine to a wider audience.

The biggest limitation of our study is the small sample size. However, the high percentage of HIV positive patients and the significant percentage of HSIL and SCC in our sample highlights the importance of regular follow up, as well as screening, especially in high-risk patients. It also illustrates the gap in preventive strategies and immunization in the male population. The need for further studies and high-level evidence in the management of CA and especially in the prevention of malignant transformation is indisputable.

Another important element regarding management of CA is high clinical suspicion. Physicians must be aware of the prevalence of this condition, the age-groups and other population sub-groups that are mostly affected, and its possible clinical manifestations. This verrucous hyperplasia can often be misdiagnosed due to its clinical presentation as multiple growths on the skin or mucous membranes [25]. They can often present also as papular to cauliflower-like lesions or as flat papular growths or as exophytic fronds [25]. Several other conditions, such as malignant lesions of the vulva, Paget's disease of the anogenital region, molluscum contagiosum, psoriasis, acrochordon, sebaceous cysts, Buschke-Lowenstein tumors, secondary syphilis, seborrheic dermatosis, popular lichen planus, and even hemorrhoids, can make the differential diagnosis challenging [1,25,26].

Final diagnosis, however, is set only after excision of the lesions through biopsy and histopathological examination. Serology tools and methodologies, including polymerase chain reaction (PCR) detection and DNA detection assays, are not considered to be reliable with an estimated level of evidence of 2b. Moreover, it is not possible to have cultures of the virus. While the sample that can be used to detect the virus using PCR can be the same as the one used for cytological examination, several limitations are present regarding these methods. Most of the time, only a small sample is obtained, which can lead to sampling errors even when very sensitive assays are used. Another limitation concerns the menstrual cycle, which can also tamper with serology and molecular results [27,28]. Molecular diagnostic techniques for detection of HPV, although available, are not used as a standard screening procedure as it is believed that they would overestimate the proportion of women who have low-grade cytological abnormalities and do not also meet the criteria for a secondary prevention method (screening) [28,29]. Limitations also include the fact that various HPV genotypes can be present in each patient, while HPV persistence has been also identified as a key factor as a specific subtype cannot always be easy to identify. Therefore, the clinical utility of these serology and molecular HPV diagnostic tools requires careful management and evaluation. Overall, the adequate classification of patients into high- and low-risk groups requires accurate HPV mapping, underlying the need for further research in the domain of routine HPV molecular and serology detection [28].

Most HPV infections are subclinical and are usually handled and resolved by the immune system. HPV types can be further subcategorized to mucosal and cutaneous types. Mucosal types affect mucous membranes causing anogenital warts and neoplasia of the cervix. The squamous epithelium of the skin is infected by the cutaneous types, causing all forms of common warts, which can lead to CA. When specific oncogenic types of HPV are involved, the infected patient may develop cervical, oropharyngeal, anal, vulvar, vaginal cancer, and cancer of the penis [6,7,30].

While malignant potential and evolution to cancer strongly depends on the HPV type there are other risk factors that make certain patients more prone to an invasive type of cancer. These co-factors include mainly smoking, which seems to increase the risk of progression to high-grade dysplasia of the existing lesions, and presence of HIV infection. Immunosuppression caused by HIV significantly affects the behavior of HPV-related tumors as well as the outcome of those patients, findings that were confirmed also by the results of our cohort. The expected clearance of HPV from the immune system is significantly reduced in patients with HIV. Therefore HIV-positive patients develop HPV-related malignancies such as CA which tend to be more aggressive at a younger age and at an advanced stage upon diagnosis compared to HIV-negative patients [6]. Another important element regarding immunosuppressed individuals is that infection with LR-HPV subtypes can also lead to intraepithelial neoplasia through multiple infections which cannot be handled by the immune system [31]. In addition, in patients with genital warts and HIV infection, a greater resistance to standard treatment is observed [32].

The optimal management of CA varies depending on the lesions' size and location, but it usually includes surgical excision combined with another non-invasive technique

(Figure 8). These techniques include electrocautery ablation, laser, photodynamic therapy, carbon dioxide (CO_2), argon plasma coagulation, cryotherapy, local hyperthermia, and some medications [27,33–35]. Interestingly enough, medications that have been investigated for the treatment of CA include topical creams, such as 5-aminolevulinic acid (ALA), imiquimod 3.5%, and 5% trichloroacetic acid, podophyllotoxin, sinecatechins, and 5-fluorouracil [27,33–37]. Injection of Vitamin D3 has also been reported to achieve complete clearance of CA [38,39]. Several of these methods are used in combinations rather than as monotherapy. These not so commonly known techniques are usually being used as a curative alternative to conventional therapy methods in areas of the perineum where surgical excision is not a preferable option (e.g., penis, vulva) [33,36]. In cases of relapse, a surgeon might be left with the option of abdominoperineal resection, as presented in the results of our study (Figure 9).

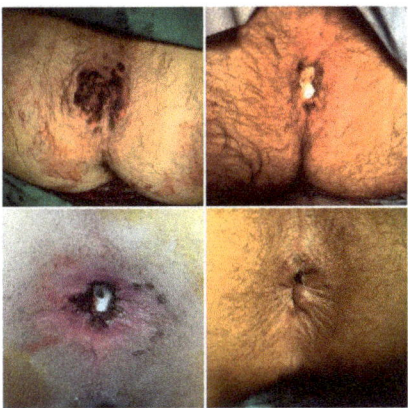

Figure 8. Final results after surgical excision of several CA lesions combined with electrocautery ablation, ultrasound scissors and diathermy.

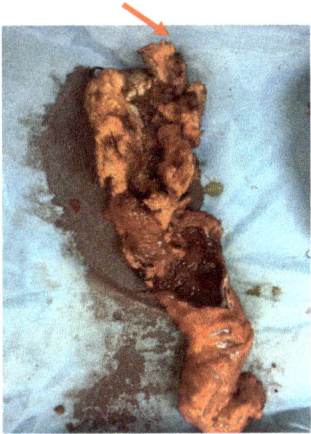

Figure 9. Specimen of abdominoperineal resection showing malignant transformation after local recurrence.

While effective in removing the skin lesions, these treatment options do not offer a chance to eradicate HPV from the human body. While macroscopical lesions can be removed effectively and often without leaving any invaded margins, HPV cannot be cleared out from the human body. This leads to the realization that it is possible to have relapses and reoccurrence of HPV-related lesions whenever certain risk factors are present and/or the immune system appears more vulnerable. Important research has been conducted in order for immunotherapy to be established as a high-efficacy treatment option. Towards this direction, Mastutik et. al. studied protein p16INK4A expression, which seems to be highly related to HR-HPV infection and may serve as a biomarker for the prediction of malignancy potential in CA lesions [40].

While the eradication of HPV infection and HPV-related lesions especially in individuals with risk factors is far from available, the need for prevention must be underlined. Primary prevention through immunization is already applicable to young girls aged 10 years (e.g., Portugal) and older requiring two or three vaccination doses based on the age of first vaccination, although most national vaccination guidelines suggest a three-dose immunization scheme [29,41]. The real controversy is whether immunization should be made available to young males and male adults. A gender-neutral vaccination program was initially doubted by the vast majority of the global community as non-cost effective. Although the available data and sample of studies are limited, there is not yet a clear path towards the ideal strategy as nearly half of the available studies are in favor of expanding immunization to young boys. Nevertheless, it is advisable that countries make decisions after carrying out further studies based on the specific national epidemiological characteristics [42]. Secondary prevention poses also a very important role mostly in women, including screening with colposcopy and vaginal cytological smear examination. Examination of the perineum will reveal not only vaginal and cervical lesions, but also anal and perianal alterations of the squamous epithelium. Finally, tertiary prevention should not be discouraged: management of precancerous HPV-related lesions in early stages using surgical excision and biopsy provides individualized treatment and can positively affect the patient's final outcome [29].

5. Conclusions

HPV remains one of the most frequently encountered STIs worldwide. Although important progress has been made in terms of preventing virus transmission through vaccine immunization, the virus remains untraceable in many cases. CA, as the clinical manifestation of HPV, affects a notable percentage of the population, especially young people. At this point, high clinical suspicion is required from all clinical doctors as CA has more treatment options and better prognosis if treated early. A delay in diagnosis can lead to malignant transformation, often leaving abdominoperineal resection as the only option. This study, although small in terms of the sample considered, aims to shed light on CA's prevalence and patients' special characteristics in a European country where not much data on the matter are available at the moment. Nevertheless, more studies are required in order to fully understand and target the most vulnerable population subgroups, raise awareness, and generalize the prevention of CA through immunization.

Author Contributions: Conceptualization, C.K. (Christoforos Kosmidis) and I.K.; methodology, C.S. and V.M.; investigation, C.S., V.M., I.C., P.R., M.D. and K.P.; writing—original draft preparation, C.S. and V.M.; writing—review and editing: C.S., C.K. (Charilaos Koulouris) and N.V.; visualization: V.T. and C.M.M.; supervision, C.K. (Christoforos Kosmidis) and I.K. All authors have read and agreed to the published version of the manuscript.

Funding: This research received no external funding.

Institutional Review Board Statement: The study was conducted in accordance with the Declaration of Helsinki, and approved by the Institutional Review Board of AHEPA University General Hospital of Thessaloniki (protocol code 8541.09.02.23).

Informed Consent Statement: Informed consent was obtained from all subjects involved in the study.

Data Availability Statement: Not applicable.

Conflicts of Interest: The authors declare no conflict of interest.

References

1. Pennycook, K.B.; McCready, T.A. Condyloma Acuminata. Available online: https://www.ncbi.nlm.nih.gov/books/NBK547667/ (accessed on 8 November 2022).
2. Sasaki, A.; Nakajima, T.; Egashira, H.; Takeda, K.; Tokoro, S.; Ichita, C.; Masuda, S.; Uojima, H.; Koizumi, K.; Kinbara, T.; et al. Condyloma acuminatum of the anal canal, treated with endoscopic submucosal dissection. *World J. Gastroenterol.* **2016**, *22*, 2636–2641. [CrossRef]
3. Rosen, T. Condylomata Acumunata (Anogenital Warts) in Adults: Epidemiology, Pathogenesis, Clinical Features, and Diagnosis. Available online: https://www.uptodate.com/contents/condylomata-acuminata-anogenital-warts-in-adults-epidemiology-pathogenesis-clinical-features-and-diagnosis#H1324464671 (accessed on 8 November 2022).
4. Clanner-Engelshofen, B.M.; Marsela, E.; Engelsberger, N.; Guertler, A.; Schauber, J.; French, L.E.; Reinholz, M. Condylomata acuminata: A retrospective analysis on clinical characteristics and treatment options. *Heliyon* **2020**, *6*, e03547. [CrossRef]
5. Leslie, S.W.; Sajjad, H.; Kumar, S. Genital Warts. Available online: https://www.ncbi.nlm.nih.gov/books/NBK441884/ (accessed on 9 November 2022).
6. Brianti, P.; De Flammineis, E.; Mercuri, S.R. Review of HPV-related diseases and cancers. *New Microbiol.* **2017**, *40*, 80–85.
7. Forcier, M.; Musacchio, N. An overview of human papillomavirus infection for the dermatologist: Disease, diagnosis, management, and prevention. *Dermatol. Ther.* **2010**, *23*, 458–476. [CrossRef]
8. Dong, Z.; Hu, R.; Du, Y.; Tan, L.; Li, L.; Du, J.; Bai, L.; Ma, Y.; Cui, H. Immunodiagnosis and Immunotherapeutics Based on Human Papillomavirus for HPV-Induced Cancers. *Front. Immunol.* **2021**, *11*, 586796. [CrossRef]
9. Doorbar, J.; Quint, W.; Banks, L.; Bravo, I.G.; Stoler, M.; Broker, T.R.; Stanley, M.A. The biology and life-cycle of human papillomaviruses. *Vaccine* **2012**, *30* (Suppl. S5), F55–F70. [CrossRef]
10. Dunne, E.F.; Park, I.U. HPV and HPV-associated diseases. *Infect. Dis. Clin. N. Am.* **2013**, *27*, 765–778. [CrossRef]
11. Schiffman, M.; Clifford, G.; Buonaguro, F.M. Classification of weakly carcinogenic human papillomavirus types: Addressing the limits of epidemiology at the borderline. *Infect. Agent Cancer* **2009**, *4*, 8. [CrossRef]
12. Berman, T.A.; Schiller, J.T. Human papillomavirus in cervical cancer and oropharyngeal cancer: One cause, two diseases. *Cancer* **2017**, *123*, 2219–2229. [CrossRef]
13. Lebreton, M.; Carton, I.; Brousse, S.; Lavoué, V.; Body, G.; Levêque, J.; Nyangoh-Timoh, K. Vulvar intraepithelial neoplasia: Classification, epidemiology, diagnosis, and management. *J. Gynecol. Obstet. Hum. Reprod.* **2020**, *49*, 101801. [CrossRef]
14. HPVirus Website. HPV Immunisation in Greece—HPV Vaccine. 2022. Available online: https://hpvcentre.net/statistics/reports/GRC.pdf (accessed on 8 November 2022).
15. Irshad, U.; Puckett, Y. *Giant Condylomata Acuminata of Buschke and Lowenstein*; StatPearls: Treasure Island, FL, USA, 2022.
16. Davis, K.G.; Barton, J.S.; Orangio, G.; Bivin, W.; Krane, S. Buschke-Lowenstein Tumors: A Review and Proposed Classification System. *Sex. Transm. Dis.* **2021**, *48*, e263–e268. [CrossRef]
17. Furukawa, S.; Uota, S.; Yamana, T.; Sahara, R.; Iihara, K.; Yokomaku, Y.; Iwatani, Y.; Sugiura, W. Distribution of Human Papillomavirus Genotype in Anal Condyloma Acuminatum Among Japanese Men: The Higher Prevalence of High Risk Human Papillomavirus in Men Who Have Sex with Men with HIV Infection. *AIDS Res. Hum. Retrovir.* **2018**, *34*, 375–381. [CrossRef] [PubMed]
18. Hagensee, M.E.; Cameron, J.E.; Leigh, J.E.; Clark, R.A. Human papillomavirus infection and disease in HIV-infected individuals. *Am. J. Med. Sci.* **2004**, *328*, 57–63. [CrossRef]
19. Arnold, J.D.; Byrne, M.E.; Monroe, A.K.; Abbott, S.E.; District of Columbia Cohort Executive Committee. The Risk of Anal Carcinoma after Anogenital Warts in Adults Living with HIV. *JAMA Dermatol.* **2021**, *157*, 283–289. [CrossRef]
20. Albuquerque, A.; Cappello, C.; Stirrup, O. High-risk human papilloma virus, pre-cancerous lesions and cancer in anal warts. *AIDS* **2021**, *35*, 1939–1948. [CrossRef] [PubMed]
21. Burd, E.M. Human papillomavirus and cervical cancer. *Clin. Microbiol. Rev.* **2003**, *16*, 1–17. [CrossRef]
22. Park, I.U.; Introcaso, C.; Dunne, E.F. Human Papillomavirus and Genital Warts: A Review of the Evidence for the 2015 Centers for Disease Control and Prevention Sexually Transmitted Diseases Treatment Guidelines. *Clin. Infect. Dis.* **2015**, *61* (Suppl. S8), S849–S855. [CrossRef] [PubMed]
23. The ANCHOR Study Website. Available online: https://anchorstudy.org (accessed on 10 November 2022).
24. Chikandiwa, A.; Chimoyi, L.; Pisa, P.T.; Chersich, M.F.; Muller, E.E.; Michelow, P.; Mayaud, P.; Delany-Moretlwe, S. Prevalence of anogenital HPV infection, related disease and risk factors among HIV-infected men in inner-city Johannesburg, South Africa: Baseline findings from a cohort study. *BMC Public Health* **2017**, *17* (Suppl. S3), 425. [CrossRef]
25. Steben, M.; Garland, S.M. Genital Warts. *Best Pract. Res. Clin. Obstet. Gynaecol.* **2014**, *28*, 1063–1073. [CrossRef]
26. Kosmidis, C.S.; Sevva, C.; Roulia, P.; Koulouris, C.; Varsamis, N.; Koimtzis, G.; Theodorou, V.; Mystakidou, C.M.; Georgakoudi, E.; Anthimidis, G. Extramammary Paget's Disease of the Vulva: Report of Two Cases. *Medicina* **2021**, *57*, 1029. [CrossRef]
27. Sindhuja, T.; Bhari, N.; Gupta, S. Asian guidelines for condyloma acuminatum. *J. Infect. Chemother.* **2022**, *28*, 845–852. [CrossRef]
28. Molijn, A.; Kleter, B.; Quint, W.; van Doorn, L.J. Molecular diagnosis of human papillomavirus (HPV) infections. *J. Clin. Virol.* **2005**, *32* (Suppl. S1), S43–S51. [CrossRef] [PubMed]
29. Adams, T.S.; Rogers, L.J.; Cuello, M.A. Cancer of the vagina: 2021 update. *Int. J. Gynaecol. Obstet.* **2021**, *155* (Suppl. S1), 19–27. [CrossRef] [PubMed]

30. Giannaki, M.; Kakourou, T.; Theodoridou, M.; Syriopoulou, V.; Kabouris, M.; Louizou, E.; Chrousos, G. Human papillomavirus (HPV) genotyping of cutaneous warts in Greek children. *Pediatr. Dermatol.* **2013**, *30*, 730–735. [CrossRef] [PubMed]
31. Kreuter, A.; Siorokos, C.; Oellig, F.; Silling, S.; Pfister, H.; Wieland, U. High-grade Dysplasia in Anogenital Warts of HIV-Positive Men. *JAMA Dermatol.* **2016**, *152*, 1225–1230. [CrossRef]
32. Reusser, N.M.; Downing, C.; Guidry, J.; Tyring, S.K. HPV Carcinomas in Immunocompromised Patients. *J. Clin. Med.* **2015**, *4*, 260–281. [CrossRef]
33. Yin, G.; Zhang, Y.; Geng, M.; Cai, B.; Zheng, Y. Cure of condyloma acuminata covering the glans penis using aminolevulinic acid/photodynamic therapy. *Photodiagn. Photodyn. Ther.* **2020**, *30*, 101658. [CrossRef]
34. Sugai, S.; Nishijima, K.; Enomoto, T. Management of Condyloma Acuminata in Pregnancy: A Review. *Sex. Transm. Dis.* **2021**, *48*, 403–409. [CrossRef]
35. Yin, G.; Sha, K.; Cai, B.; Li, F.; Li, X.; Xia, X.; Pan, X. Effect of 5-aminolevulinic acid photodynamic therapy on keratinocyte proliferation and apoptosis in condyloma acuminatum. *Photodiagn. Photodyn. Ther.* **2017**, *18*, 310–314. [CrossRef]
36. Hum, M.; Chow, E.; Schuurmans, N.; Dytoc, M. Case of giant vulvar condyloma acuminata successfully treated with imiquimod 3.75% cream: A case report. *SAGE Open Med. Case Rep.* **2018**, *6*, 2050313X18802143. [CrossRef]
37. Celayir, M.F.; Kartal, K.; Mihmanli, M. A comparative study of two techniques in the treatment of condyloma acuminata. *Ann. Ital. Chir.* **2018**, *89*, 455–460.
38. Jha, N. Complete clearance of condyloma acuminata using injection Vitamin D3. *Australas. J. Dermatol.* **2021**, *62*, e417–e418. [CrossRef] [PubMed]
39. Rind, T.; Oiso, N.; Kawada, A. Successful Treatment of Anogenital Wart with a Topical Vitamin D(3) Derivative in an Infant. *Case Rep. Dermatol.* **2010**, *2*, 46–49. [CrossRef] [PubMed]
40. Mastutik, G.; Rahniayu, A.; Arista, A.; Murtiastutik, D.; Kurniasari, N.; Setyaningrum, T.; Rahaju, A.S.; Sulistyani, E. p16INK4A Expression in Condyloma Acuminata Lesions Associated with High-Risk Human Papillomavirus Infection. *Asian Pac. J. Cancer Prev.* **2021**, *22*, 3219–3225. [CrossRef] [PubMed]
41. Margolis, M.A.; Brewer, N.T.; Shah, P.D.; Calo, W.A.; Alton Dailey, S.; Gilkey, M.B. Talking about recommended age or fewer doses: What motivates HPV vaccination timeliness? *Hum. Vaccin. Immunother.* **2021**, *17*, 3077–3080. [CrossRef]
42. Linertová, R.; Guirado-Fuentes, C.; Mar Medina, J.; Imaz-Iglesia, I.; Rodríguez-Rodríguez, L.; Carmona-Rodríguez, M. Cost-effectiveness of extending the HPV vaccination to boys: A systematic review. *J. Epidemiol. Community Health* **2021**, *75*, 910–916. [CrossRef] [PubMed]

Disclaimer/Publisher's Note: The statements, opinions and data contained in all publications are solely those of the individual author(s) and contributor(s) and not of MDPI and/or the editor(s). MDPI and/or the editor(s) disclaim responsibility for any injury to people or property resulting from any ideas, methods, instructions or products referred to in the content.

Endometrial Staining of CD56 (Uterine Natural Killer), BCL-6, and CD138 (Plasma Cells) Improve Diagnosis and Clinical Pregnancy Outcomes in Unexplained Infertility and Recurrent IVF Failures: Standardization of Diagnosis with Digital Pathology

Suheyla Ekemen [1,2,*], Cem Comunoglu [3], Cavit Kerem Kayhan [2], Ebru Bilir [4], Ilkay Cavusoglu [5], Nilay Etiler [6,7], Selcuk Bilgi [2], Umit Ince [2,8], Cevayir Coban [9,*] and Halit Firat Erden [10,†]

1. Vocational School of Health Services, Kerem Aydınlar Campus, Acıbadem University, Istanbul 34752, Turkey
2. Acıbadem Central Pathology Laboratory, Kerem Aydinlar Campus, Istanbul 34752, Turkey
3. Department of Pathology, Dr. Cemil Tascioglu City Hospital, University of Health Sciences, Istanbul 34668, Turkey
4. School of Medicine, Bahcesehir University, Istanbul 34349, Turkey
5. Women's Health and Gynecological Nursing, Institute of Health Sciences, Biruni University, Istanbul 34010, Turkey
6. Department of Public Health, School of Medicine, Istanbul Okan University, Istanbul 34947, Turkey
7. Public Health Department, University of Nevada, Reno, NV 89509, USA
8. Department of Digital Pathology, School of Medicine, Acıbadem University, Istanbul 34752, Turkey
9. Division of Malaria Immunology, Department of Microbiology and Immunology, Institute of Medical Science (IMSUT), University of Tokyo, Tokyo 108-8639, Japan
10. Obstetrics and Gynecology Infertility Clinic, Zorlu Center, Istanbul 34340, Turkey

* Correspondence: suheylaekemen@gmail.com (S.E.); ccoban@ims.u-tokyo.ac.jp (C.C.)
† Deceased.

Abstract: In women with unexplained infertility (UI) and recurrent in vitro fertilization (IVF) failures, the etiology is often unclear. Endometrial immune perturbations and the use of immune markers associated with these dysregulations are of great interest in the diagnosis and treatment of UI. However, reliable biomarkers and standardized quantification methods are lacking. Here, to address endometrial immune dysregulation in UI patients with recurrent IVF failures, we performed endometrial tissue sampling and immunostaining of CD56 (uNK), CD138, and BCL-6. Of these cases, 57.9% had positive CD56 in the endometrial stroma, while 46.1% had positive BCL-6 in the glandular epithelium, and 14.5% of the cases were found to be positive for CD138. Combined staining rates were 60.5%, 68.4%, and 71.05% for (CD56 or BCL-6), (CD56 or CD138), and (CD56, BCL-6, or CD138), respectively. There was a significant correlation between CD56 and BCL-6 positivity, while CD138 positivity was an independent parameter. After the recommended targeted therapy, pregnancy rates were found to increase from 58.5% to 61.6% and 73.8% in CD56-positive, (CD56- or BCL-6-positive), and (CD56-, BCL-6-, or CD138-positive) cases, respectively. Notably, a retrospective evaluation of digital pathology and light microscopy results showed a significant correlation. This study suggests that the examination of CD56, BCL-6, and CD138 in the same endometrial sample may be an effective method in determining the etiology of UI and reaching an early diagnosis and treatment options. Moreover, digital pathology can be used in the evaluation of CD56 and BCL-6 to provide objective, rapid, and reliable results.

Keywords: unexplained infertility (UI); recurrent IVF failures; endometriosis; endometritis; CD56 (uNK); BCL-6; CD138

1. Introduction

Unexplained infertility (UI) is defined after normal results of intensive infertility evaluation and accounts for approximately 15–30% of infertility cases [1]. In vitro fertilization (IVF) is used in cases of UI; however, recurrent IVF failures are common [2]. Endometriosis is thought to be among the significant causes of UI. However, laparoscopic diagnosis of endometriosis may not be accurate [3], and accurate diagnosis is important for successful treatment outcomes [3,4]. In recent years, the use of immune markers that are related to changes in endometrial immunity and microbiota and the detection of immune disruption of the endometrium have received considerable attention in the diagnosis, staging, and treatment of UI [5–7]. However, there are no standardized criteria on how to objectively assess and validate these immune markers in the endometrium.

The leukocytes in the endometrium are clearly different from those of the peripheral blood and consist mainly of uterine natural killer cells (uNK, ~70%) and other cells such as macrophages, neutrophils, mast cells, dendritic cells, and T and B cells [6,7]. The uterine NK cells express CD56 (the uNK marker, also known as the neural cell adhesion molecule), but not other classical NK cells or T-cell markers. The number of uNK cells is known to change during the menstrual cycle, pregnancy, and various pathologies of the endometrium, with controversial results. Activated uNK cells are involved in the regulation of trophoblast invasion into the decidua [8,9]. The elevation of CD56, which normally shows a slight increase in the endometrial stroma during the preimplantation period, has been found to be higher in infertile women and in pregnancy loss [2,8,10–12]. There appears to be a direct correlation between CD56 elevation and pelvic endometriosis [11,13–19].

B-cell lymphoma 6 protein (BCL-6) was first identified as an oncogene important for proliferation in B-cell lymphomas but was later found in various tumors, as well as endometrial pathologies. Several recent studies have investigated the relationship between the expression rate of BCL-6 in the endometrial gland epithelium and endometriosis [5,20–23]. Increased BCL-6 expression has been shown in UI and recurrent IVF failures [21,22]. BCL-6 overexpression has been associated with increased cellular proliferation [24]. A high expression of BCL-6 in women with endometriosis has been associated with a decrease in progesterone activating and regulating receptors and the inactivation of progesterone in the endometrium [22]. BCL-6 is thought to be responsible for progesterone resistance in the endometrium of women with endometriosis [20,22,23]. BCL-6 is also the master regulatory gene that is essential for T follicular helper cell differentiation, as well as B cell differentiation in germinal centers (GCs), and its regulation by various factors may play a role in autoantibody development [25,26]. Therefore, an abnormal expression of endometrial BCL-6 may be responsible for poor reproductive outcomes after embryo transfer [21,27].

Chronic endometritis is an inflammation of the endometrium that prevents implantation and is another possible cause of infertility [7]. The immunohistochemical presence of plasma cells (CD138, also known as syndecan-1) in endometrial specimens is thought to be an objective diagnosis of chronic endometritis [28]. However, there is still no clear consensus on the threshold for the number of plasma cells in the endometrium and its correlation with UI, and the treatment outcomes have not been confirmed.

We hypothesized that a combination of different immune markers would be a better diagnostic approach in the endometrial material from women with UI and recurrent implantation failures. Therefore, here, we evaluated the combination of three markers (CD56, BCL-6, and CD138) in curettage material from women with UI and recurrent IVF failures. We examined the association between these biomarkers and clinical pregnancy outcomes after treatment. Digital image analysis has recently been introduced for cell density estimation of the endometrium as an easier, faster, and standardized assessment of pathology specimens [17,29,30]. Therefore, we additionally compared immunohistochemical panel assessment with light microscopy (LM) and digital pathology (DP) performed by expert pathologists in order to assess and validate the objective criteria without major diagnostic errors and to eliminate any differences between the assessments.

2. Materials and Methods

2.1. Study Population and Ethics Approval

In this retrospective study, the endometrial biopsy materials of 76 women with UI and recurrent IVF failures were included. The inclusion criteria were as follows: (i) no male infertility, (ii) no evidence of endometriosis by laparoscopic or clinical examination, (iii) no laboratory evidence of acute infections, such as HCV, HBV, HIV, or Rubella, and (iv) no abnormal serum prolactin, T3, T4, FSH, LH, Estradiol (E2), and progesterone (P4) levels. The women were aged 23–45 years (33.7± 4.5, mean ± SD), had no previous pregnancies, and had experienced at least one, and up to 8, IVF failures (Table 1). After IVF, all of the women were routinely followed up for successful clinical pregnancy outcomes with serum beta-hCG (10–11 days after implantation) and ultrasound (presence of gestational sac and the fetal heartbeat investigated 4–5 weeks after implantation). A total of 65.8% of the women were aged 30–39 years, and 57.9% had 3 or more IVF failures. A total of 15.8% of the women had 5–8 IVF failures, while more than 80% had 1–4 IVF failures.

Table 1. Characteristics of the study population who were diagnosed with unexplained infertility (UI).

Characteristics	Number ($n = 76$)	Percentage (%)
Age groups		
<25	1	1.3
25–29	17	22.4
30–34	25	32.9
35–39	25	32.9
≥40	8	10.5
Number of IVF failures		
1–2	32	40.8
3–4	32	40.8
5–6	10	15.8
7–8	2	2.6

Ethical approval was obtained from Acibadem University Faculty of Medicine Ethics Committee (ATADEK2019-1/14).

2.2. Endometrial Sampling and Immunostaining

Endometrial sampling was performed in the secretory phase between days 22 and 23 of the cycle after daily monitoring of endometrial thickness by ultrasound and blood hormone levels every other day. All samples were fixed in 10% neutral-buffered formalin solution and processed with a Tissue-Tek Vip® 6 AI device (Sakura Finetek Japan Co., Ltd., Tokyo, Japan) [31] to prepare paraffin blocks. Three-µm-thick sections were prepared from all of the blocks and stained with hematoxylin and eosin (H&E) using a Shandon Gemini stainer. Immunohistochemical staining was performed using antibodies against CD56 (CD564 clone, Leica Biosystems, Wetzlar, Germany), CD138 (B-A38 clone, Biocare Medical, Pacheco, CA, USA), and BCL-6 (LN 22 clone, Biocare Medical, Pacheco, CA, USA) using a Ventana Benchmark XT device (Roche Diagnostics, Basel, Switzerland).

2.3. Evaluation by Conventional Light Microscopy (LM)

All of the slides were morphologically evaluated and reported by two independent pathologists (S.E. and C.Com.) who were experienced in the field of gynecological pathology using a light microscope (LM) (Olympus BX51). CD56+ cells in the stroma were assessed on a semiquantitative scale as a percentage of the endometrial stromal cells, where a reference value of more than 6% was established (<6% is considered negative and ≥6% is considered positive staining). For CD138 staining, two independent pathologists screened the entire slide (~100 × 80 mm² area) and the entire stroma section at ×400 magnification, and ≥1 plasma cell was considered to be a positive value [32]. The number of CD138-positive plasma cells ranged from 7 to 121 cells (53.7 ± 41.4, mean ± SD) in positive cases.

BCL-6+ cells in the glandular region were assessed using the proposed HSCORE (0–4) system to minimize the difference between the observers [5,33]. Briefly, the HSCORE was calculated as the membranous staining intensity of BCL-6 in glandular cells (absent: 0, weak: 1, moderate: 2, and strong: 3) and the epsilon value was obtained by dividing the sum of the product of the individual gland percentages by 100, with the formula HSCORE = $\sum Pi\ (I + 1)/100$ (i = staining intensities and Pi = the percentage of stained cells for each intensity, ranging from 0% to 100%) [5]. An HSCORE reference value of ≥ 1.4 was considered positive staining and <1.4 was considered to be a negative BCL-6 value. Neuroendocrine tumor sections for CD56 and lymph node sections for BCL-6 and CD138 were used as positive controls.

2.4. Digital Pathology (DP)

In addition to the conventional pathology reports, the same slides were re-evaluated with the 3DHISTECH CaseViewer program (3DHISTECH Ltd., The Digital Pathology Company, Budapest, Hungary), a digital microscopy application designed to support the histopathologic diagnosis and microscopy review process at Acibadem University, which has been used since 2014 [34]. As with conventional light microscopy, CD56 positivity was calculated as a percentage in stromal cells. BCL-6 staining in the glandular epithelium was, to our knowledge, digitally calculated for the first time in this study using the HSCORE (0–4) scoring system. Since we considered ≥ 1 plasma cell positivity with LM as positive-CD138 staining, and a sign of chronic endometritis, we did not evaluate CD138 positivity with DP separately.

2.5. Statistical Analysis

All statistical analyses were performed with IBM SPSS (Statistical Package for the Social Sciences) version 28 (IBM Corp., Armonk, NY, USA). Associations between continuous data were tested using Pearson's correlation tests. In all analyses, the statistical significance level (p-value) was considered to be less than 0.05.

3. Results

3.1. Immunopathology Detection of the Endometrium by Conventional Light Microscopy

A total of 76 women aged 23–45 years (33.7 ± 4.5, mean ± SD) with at least one, and up to eight, IVF failures were included in this study after careful exclusion of other factors, such as male infertility, infections, endometriosis, and hormonal abnormalities (Table 1). CD56 positivity in the endometrial stroma by LM was calculated as <6% (negative) and $\geq 6\%$ (positive) (Figure 1A). A total of 44 (57.9%) cases had values of 6% or more for CD56 immunostaining in the endometrial stroma, while 35 cases (46%) had an HSCORE of 1.4 or higher for BCL-6 immunostaining in the glandular epithelium (Figure 1B and Table 2), and 11 cases (14.5%) were positive for CD138 staining and were considered to be chronic endometritis (Figure 1C). Corresponding H&E sections and positive controls are shown in Figure 1D,E, respectively.

Two or more IVF failures occurred in 74.3% of CD56+ cases and 65.7% of BCL-6+ cases. It is noteworthy that 75% of those CD56+ cases (33 out of 44) had BCL-6 HSCORE values above 1.4 in the glandular epithelium. Pearson's correlation test revealed a moderate but significant correlation between CD56 and BCL-6 positivity, with r = 0.576 and $p < 0.001$ (Table 3). In contrast, among the CD138+ cases, CD56 positivity was observed in only two cases (18.2%) and BCL-6 positivity in only one case (9%). Therefore, we considered CD138 positivity as an independent, but additional, endometrial marker for the immune pathology of the endometrium, i.e., chronic endometritis. On the other hand, when combined, CD56 and BCL-6 positivity increased to 60.5%, while the overall detection of endometrial pathology with the combination of CD56, BCL-6, and CD138 was 71.05% (Table 2). Twenty-two cases (28.9%) did not show positive immunostaining with any marker.

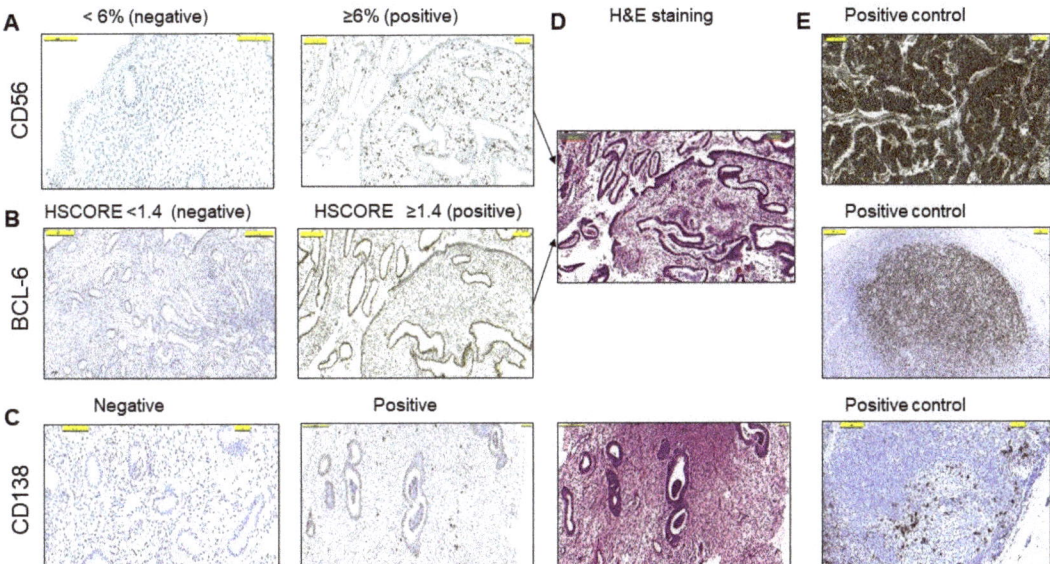

Figure 1. The semiquantitative analysis of the endometrium by conventional light microscopy (LM). (**A**) Representative examples of positive (≥6%) and negative (<6%) cells with immunohistochemical staining for CD56 in the stroma. (**B**) Representative examples of HSCORE grading of positive (≥1.4) and negative (<1.4) cells with immunohistochemical staining for BCL-6 in the glandular epithelium. (**C**) Representative examples of CD138 positivity and negativity in the stroma. (**D**) H&E staining of corresponding positive IHC sections in (**A–C**). (**E**) Irrelevant neuroendocrine tumor section in A and lymph node sections in B and C were used as positive controls. The pictures are at the same magnification.

Table 2. The rates of clinical pregnancy outcome by immune markers.

Immune Markers	Definition	Positivity Rate $n = 76$ (%)	Clinical Pregnancy Outcome $n = 65$ (%)
CD56 Levels	≥6%	44 (57.9)	38 (58.5%)
BCL-6 Levels	HSCORE ≥ 1.4	35 (46.1)	30 (46.2%)
CD56 or BCL-6	CD56 ≥ 6% or BCL-6 HSCORE ≥ 1.4	46 (60.5)	40 (61.5%)
CD56 or CD138	CD56 ≥ 6% or CD138 ≥ 1	52 (68.4)	46 (70.8%)
CD56, BCL-6, or CD138	CD56 ≥ 6%, BCL-6 HSCORE ≥ 1.4, or CD138 ≥ 1	54 (71.05)	48 (73.8%)

Table 3. Correlations of CD56 and BCL-6 immunohistochemical markers with light microscopy (LM) and digital pathology (DP).

	Correlation Coefficient (r)	p *
CD56 (LM) vs. CD56 (DP)	0.906	<0.001
BCL-6 (LM) vs. BCL-6 (DP)	0.943	<0.001
CD56 (LM) vs. BCL-6 (LM)	0.576	<0.001
CD56 (DP) vs. BCL-6 (DP)	0.592	<0.001

LM: Light microscopy, DP: Digital pathology. * Pearson's correlation test.

3.2. Targeted Treatment Based on Immune Marker Detection Increased Pregnancy Rates

After examining the cases with immunohistochemistry, the infertility center was advised to use CD56 positivity $\geq 6\%$ and BCL-6 HSCORE ≥ 1.4 as references for the treatment options based on the previous literature [5,17]. When the CD56 reference value exceeded the positivity criteria ($\geq 6\%$), the patients were treated with cortisone and/or intralipid therapy [16,35]. A high BCL-6 HSCORE is generally used to detect both occult endometriosis and the development of progesterone resistance [20]. However, due to the higher levels of BCL-6 and CD56 positivity together, 94.3% of the BCL-6+ cases were treated similarly to the CD56+ cases, except for one patient who refused treatment despite double positivity with BCL-6 and CD56. In addition, any positive value for CD138 staining in the endometrial stroma was considered to be chronic endometritis and received antibiotic treatment [36]. The cases without positivity for any of the studied markers were evaluated for other options.

Finally, we followed the patients for clinical pregnancy success and compared them with the immune marker results in the pathology report. Clinical pregnancy was routinely assessed by monitoring serum beta-hCG levels and ultrasonographic evaluation for the presence of a gestational sac and fetal heartbeat. Overall, successful pregnancy outcomes were achieved in 85.5% of cases (65 out of 76 cases). We then evaluated the contribution of single and/or combined immunostaining results to successful clinical pregnancy outcomes. Single positive staining with CD56, BCL-6, or CD138 showed relatively higher clinical pregnancy rates (58.5%, 46.2%, and 16.9%, respectively). However, the highest pregnancy success occurred in the total cluster of cases staining positive for CD56, BCL-6, or CD138 markers, with 73.8% of clinical pregnancies occurring in this group (Table 2). On the other hand, the group in which all of the markers were negative (comprising 28.9% of all cases) contributed only 26.5% of the successful clinical pregnancy rates. Together, these results suggest that increased numbers of immune marker detection, followed by targeted therapy, significantly improve clinical pregnancy rates.

3.3. Digital Pathology Analysis of CD56 and BCL-6 Immunostaining of the Endometrium

We then evaluated the same slides using the DP setting of the 3DHISTECH Case-Viewer program, which has been installed, optimized, and routinely used at Acibadem University since 2014 [34]. The criteria for CD56 or BCL-6 positivity did not differ from the conventional microscopy evaluation methodology, but this time the evaluation was performed with DP (Figure 2A). Similar to the LM results, DP yielded values of 6% or higher for CD56 immunostaining in the endometrial stroma in 44 cases (57.9%), and HSCORE values of 1.4 or higher for BCL-6 immunostaining in the glandular epithelium in 35 cases (46%) (Figure 2B).

To investigate the value of DP over conventional microscopy, we compared the LM assessment results of both CD56 and BCL-6 with the DP results. There was a statistically strong correlation between the CD56 values measured by LM and DP ($r = 0.90$, $p < 0.001$, by Pearson's correlation test). There was also a high correlation between the HSCORE values of the BCL-6 assessed by LM and the BCL-6 assessed by DP ($r = 0.94$, $p < 0.001$, by Pearson's correlation test) (Table 3). In addition, a significant correlation between CD56 and BCL-6 positivity with both LM and DP ($r = 0.576$, $p < 0.001$ and $r = 0.592$, $p < 0.001$, respectively, by Pearson correlation test) was observed (Table 3). Furthermore, when the LM results of the CD138 levels were added, the percentage of endometrial pathology diagnosed by DP reached 69.7%, comparable to the LM analysis.

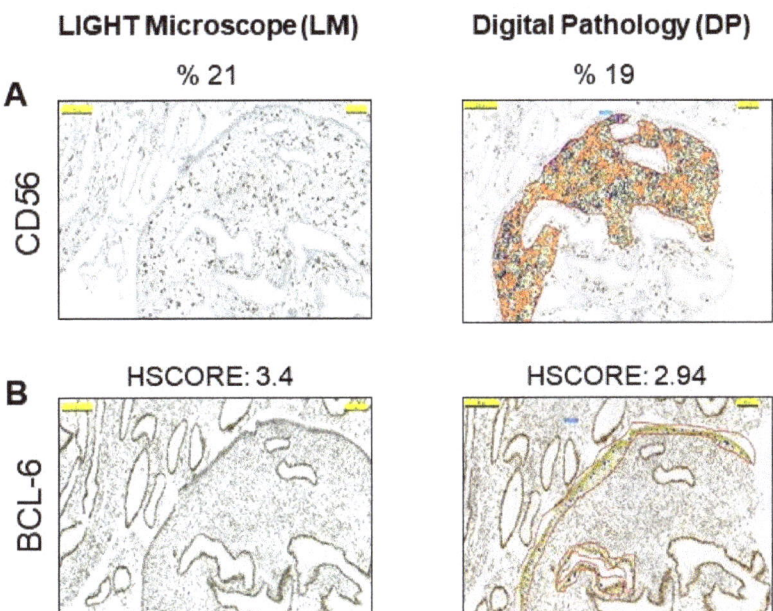

Figure 2. Digital pathology analysis of the endometrium by 3DHISTECH CaseViewer. (**A**) Representative examples of positive cells with digital imaging for CD56 in the stroma. (**B**) Representative examples of HSCORE grading of positive cells with digital imaging for BCL-6 in glandular epithelium. The pictures are at the same magnification.

4. Discussion

Endometrial immune dysregulation is well recognized as a cause of UI and recurrent IVF failure; however, there is no consensus on which biomarkers or standard diagnostic criteria should be evaluated. Here, we found that a combination of immunohistochemical staining of the endometrial stroma with uNK cell marker CD56 and the plasma cell marker CD138, together with BCL-6 immunostaining of the glandular epithelium in sections of the same specimen, can significantly improve the diagnostic and therapeutic outcomes of UI and IVF failures. Notably, the evaluation of three different immunostains can be reliably standardized using digital pathology, which enables the quick, easy, and objective evaluation of specimens.

Previous studies have shown that, apart from physiological endometrial cycles [2], CD56 levels in the endometrial stroma can also be elevated when immunological disturbances occur in the endometrium, and recurrent implantation failures may occur due to cytokine release from these CD56+ uNK cells [2,11–13,17,18,37]. In this study, we found that the CD56 levels were highly elevated in the endometrial stroma of most women (57.9%) with UI and recurrent IVF failure. Although there is no clear reference value for determining CD56 levels [10], the use of cortisone and/or intravenous intralipid has been recommended when CD56 positivity is above 6%, based on the previous reports [16,38]. Therefore, the infertility center was guided to set the reference value as $\geq 6\%$ CD56 positivity for the treatment decision and follow-up. According to the LM review by two independent pathologists, 44 cases with high CD56 levels were treated with cortisone and/or intralipid, and pregnancy occurred in 86.4% of these cases. Although calculating the percentage of CD56 positivity in the endometrial stroma with LM gives clear results, it is laborious and time consuming. Moreover, since the assessment is subjective, there may be variations between the evaluators. Our findings revealed that DP of immunopathology slides, as a new technology [39], showed a strong correlation with LM results (Table 3). Therefore, it should be considered that CD56 immunostaining can be objectively, reliably, and rapidly assessed by DP in the future.

Immunohistochemical staining of BCL-6 in the endometrium has recently emerged as a new marker to be evaluated when the cause of infertility is in question [5,20–23]. Increased staining and intensity of BCL-6 in endometrial glands has previously been associated with the identification of pelvic endometriosis[5,] where it may interfere with embryo implantation [20,22]. Therefore, the measurement of BCL-6 levels in the endometrial tissue is valuable, both for the definitive detection of endometriosis[3] and for possible progesterone resistance in the endometrium [20]. We evaluated BCL-6 levels by LM based on HSCORE scoring and found 46% positivity in our cases. We also performed, to the best of our knowledge, the first digital assessment of BCL-6 immunostaining based on HSCORE and found that DP and LM results showed a strong correlation (Table 3); however, there were also some unexpected differences. For example, in one case, although the LM assessment value was very low (HSCORE = 0.5), the digital pathology measurement was 1.6. In this case, the CD56 level in the stromal cells was calculated as 4% (below the cut-off value of <6%), therefore, the case did not receive treatment and pregnancy did not occur. Would the outcome have been different if this case had received treatment according to the high BCL-6 level that was calculated by DP? We do not know the answer to this. However, this example shows that BCL-6 assessment in LM can vary greatly depending on the interpreter. Therefore, it seems that HSCORE assessment of BCL-6 with digital pathology may be more reliable and faster.

CD138 immunostaining was positive in 14.5% of the cases, while only two cases were found to be positive with CD56 immunostaining, suggesting that there is no correlation between CD56 and CD138 positivity. Our evaluation showed that the LM assessment setting of ≥1% for CD138 positivity did not require DP evaluation. Therefore, we did not perform CD138 assessment by DP, and strongly recommend screening of immunohistochemistry sections by LM for CD138 evaluation. Nevertheless, the positive cases that were diagnosed with chronic endometritis were treated with standard antibiotic therapy [28]. Surprisingly, all 11 cases achieved pregnancy after such treatment. Although a few studies disagree with our findings [32], we recommend that CD138 immunostaining be considered as an independent marker for the evaluation of endometrial specimens. However, a larger sample size is needed in the future for a more definitive decision.

Our analysis of two and three staining procedures in the same sample showed that the percentage of endometrial perturbation diagnosis in all of the cases increased by 57.9%, 60.5%, and 71.05% for CD56, CD56 or BCL-6, and CD56, BCL-6, or CD138 positivity, respectively. Interestingly, among the immune-marker-positive cases (all but one of the case received treatment), the pregnancy rate reached 73.8% for the three-marker-stains (CD56, BCL-6, or CD138). Three-marker-negative staining was seen in only 28.9% of cases, and the contribution of this group to the successful clinical pregnancy rate was only 26.15%, well below the marker-positive and treated group. Given the limited number of cases in this group, larger studies with appropriate controls are still needed in the future for a definitive analysis.

In summary, we suggest that CD56, CD138, and BCL-6 immunomarkers should be studied together in a single session in curettage material from women with UI and recurrent IVF failure in the same cycle. In specimens with all three immunohistochemical stains, chronic endometritis (CD138) and CD56 elevation (an increase in uNK cells) can be detected first, and a specific treatment can be easily given. The secondary benefit is directed towards BCL-6. In our study, BCL-6 correlated well with CD56 positivity, even better than CD56 immunopositivity alone. In addition, since BCL-6 positivity is associated with pelvic endometriosis, immunostaining of curettage material may allow for an easy diagnosis and protect individuals from more invasive interventions. Therefore, further studies are needed in order to evaluate BCL-6 positivity in the endometrium.

5. Study Limitations

The current study lacks further interpretation due to the lack of a control group. However, our recommendation is to examine these three markers in recurrent IVF failures after UI and to use digital pathology to provide more objective quantitative data when evaluating CD56 and BCL-6.

Author Contributions: S.E., S.B. and H.F.E. designed the study. S.E., C.C. (Cem Comunoglu), S.B. and H.F.E. analyzed the cases and prepared the data. C.K.K. made the digital pathology application. S.E., U.I., E.B. and I.C. ensured the data collection and the accuracy of the information. N.E. performed the statistical analysis. C.C. (Cevayir Coban) and C.C. (Cem Comunoglu) contributed critical comments on the interpretation of the study. S.E. wrote the manuscript and revised it with the help of C.C. (Cevayir Coban). All authors have read and agreed to the published version of the manuscript.

Funding: This research received no external funding.

Institutional Review Board Statement: The study was conducted in accordance with the Declaration of Helsinki, and approved by the Institutional Ethics Committee of Acibadem University Faculty of Medicine (protocol code ATADEK2019-1/14).

Informed Consent Statement: Informed consent was obtained from all subjects involved in the study.

Data Availability Statement: The data that support the findings of this study are available at a reasonable request from the corresponding author, S.E.

Acknowledgments: This article is dedicated to the cherished memory of our friend and colleague, H.F.E., who initiated the studies described in this paper and passed away in 2017 at the age of 51. We thank H.F.E.'s wife and legal heir, Esen Erden, for her valuable contribution to gathering data. S.E. is a Clinical Fellow of the Takeda Science Foundation and greatly acknowledges educational support from them. Cevayir Coban acknowledges support from JST-CREST and AMED (JP223fa627001 and 223fa727001). All authors have read and agreed to the published version of the manuscript.

Conflicts of Interest: The authors declare no conflict of interest.

Abbreviations

BCL-6	B-cell lymphoma 6 protein
CD138	Plasma cell marker, also known as Syndecan-1
DP	Digital pathology
IVF	In vitro fertilization
LM	Light microscopy
UI	Unexplained infertility
uNK	Uterine natural killer

References

1. Quaas, A.; Dokras, A. Diagnosis and treatment of unexplained infertility. *Rev. Obstet. Gynecol.* **2008**, *1*, 69–76. [PubMed]
2. Russell, P.; Sacks, G.; Tremellen, K.; Gee, A. The distribution of immune cells and macrophages in the endometrium of women with recurrent reproductive failure. III: Further observations and reference ranges. *Pathology* **2013**, *45*, 393–401. [CrossRef] [PubMed]
3. Mettler, L.; Shukla, D.; Schollmeyer, T. Accuracy of laparoscopic diagnosis of endometriosis. *JSLS J. Soc. Laparoendosc. Surg. Soc. Laparoendosc. Surg.* **2003**, *7*, S11. [CrossRef]
4. Máté, G.; Bernstein, L.R.; Török, A.L. Endometriosis Is a Cause of Infertility. Does Reactive Oxygen Damage to Gametes and Embryos Play a Key Role in the Pathogenesis of Infertility Caused by Endometriosis? *Front. Endocrinol.* **2018**, *9*, 725. [CrossRef] [PubMed]
5. Evans-Hoeker, E.; Lessey, B.A.; Jeong, J.W.; Savaris, R.F.; Palomino, W.A.; Yuan, L.; Schammel, D.P.; Young, S.L. Endometrial BCL6 Overexpression in Eutopic Endometrium of Women with Endometriosis. *Reprod. Sci.* **2016**, *23*, 1234–1241. [CrossRef] [PubMed]
6. Tuckerman, E.; Mariee, N.; Prakash, A.; Li, T.C.; Laird, S. Uterine natural killer cells in peri-implantation endometrium from women with repeated implantation failure after IVF. *J. Reprod. Immunol.* **2010**, *87*, 60–66. [CrossRef]
7. Agostinis, C.; Mangogna, A.; Bossi, F.; Ricci, G.; Kishore, U.; Bulla, R. Uterine immunity and microbiota: A shifting paradigm. *Front. Immunol.* **2019**, *10*, 2387. [CrossRef] [PubMed]

8. Giuliani, E.; Parkin, K.L.; Lessey, B.A.; Young, S.L.; Fazleabas, A.T. Characterization of uterine NK cells in women with infertility or recurrent pregnancy loss and associated endometriosis. *Am. J. Reprod. Immunol.* **2014**, *72*, 262–269. [CrossRef]
9. Faas, M.M.; de Vos, P. Uterine NK cells and macrophages in pregnancy. *Placenta* **2017**, *56*, 44–52. [CrossRef]
10. Chen, X.; Mariee, N.; Jiang, L.; Liu, Y.; Wang, C.C.; Li, T.C.; Laird, S. Measurement of uterine natural killer cell percentage in the periimplantation endometrium from fertile women and women with recurrent reproductive failure: Establishment of a reference range. *Am. J. Obstet. Gynecol.* **2017**, *217*, 680.e1–680.e6. [CrossRef]
11. Glover, L.E.; Crosby, D.; Thiruchelvam, U.; Harmon, C.; Ni Chorcora, C.; Wingfield, M.B.; O'Farrelly, C. Uterine natural killer cell progenitor populations predict successful implantation in women with endometriosis-associated infertility. *Am. J. Reprod. Immunol.* **2018**, *79*, e12817. [CrossRef] [PubMed]
12. Kolanska, K.; Bendifallah, S.; Cohen, J.; Placais, L.; Selleret, L.; Johanet, C.; Suner, L.; Delhommeau, F.; Chabbert-Buffet, N.; Darai, E.; et al. Unexplained recurrent implantation failures: Predictive factors of pregnancy and therapeutic management from a French multicentre study. *J. Reprod. Immunol.* **2021**, *145*, 103313. [CrossRef]
13. Xu, H. Expressions of natural cytotoxicity receptor, NKG2D and NKG2D ligands in endometriosis. *J. Reprod. Immunol.* **2019**, *136*, 102615. [CrossRef] [PubMed]
14. Wu, X.-G.; Chen, J.-J.; Zhou, H.-L.; Wu, Y.; Lin, F.; Shi, J.; Wu, H.-Z.; Xiao, H.-Q.; Wang, W. Identification and Validation of the Signatures of Infiltrating Immune Cells in the Eutopic Endometrium Endometria of Women With Endometriosis. *Front. Immunol.* **2021**, *12*, 671201. [CrossRef]
15. Fukui, A.; Mai, C.; Saeki, S.; Yamamoto, M.; Takeyama, R.; Kato, T.; Ukita, Y.; Wakimoto, Y.; Yamaya, A.; Shibahara, H. Pelvic endometriosis and natural killer cell immunity. *Am. J. Reprod. Immunol.* **2020**, *85*, e13342. [CrossRef] [PubMed]
16. Fukui, A.; Kamoi, M.; Funamizu, A.; Fuchinoue, K.; Chiba, H.; Yokota, M.; Fukuhara, R.; Mizunuma, H. NK cell abnormality and its treatment in women with reproductive failures such as recurrent pregnancy loss, implantation failures, preeclampsia, and pelvic endometriosis. *Reprod. Med. Biol.* **2015**, *14*, 151–157. [CrossRef]
17. Lash, G.E.; Bulmer, J.N.; Li, T.C.; Innes, B.A.; Mariee, N.; Patel, G.; Sanderson, J.; Quenby, S.; Laird, S.M. Standardisation of uterine natural killer (uNK) cell measurements in the endometrium of women with recurrent reproductive failure. *J. Reprod. Immunol.* **2016**, *116*, 50–59. [CrossRef]
18. Freitag, N.; Pour, S.J.; Fehm, T.N.; Toth, B.; Markert, U.R.; Weber, M.; Togawa, R.; Kruessel, J.-S.; Baston-Buest, D.M.; Bielfeld, A.P. Are uterine natural killer and plasma cells in infertility patients associated with endometriosis, repeated implantation failure, or recurrent pregnancy loss? *Arch. Gynecol. Obstet.* **2020**, *302*, 1487–1494. [CrossRef]
19. Bulun, S.E.; Yilmaz, B.D.; Sison, C.; Miyazaki, K.; Bernardi, L.; Liu, S.; Kohlmeier, A.; Yin, P.; Milad, M.; Wei, J. Endometriosis. *Endocr. Rev.* **2019**, *40*, 1048–1079. [CrossRef]
20. Likes, C.E.; Cooper, L.J.; Efird, J.; Forstein, D.A.; Miller, P.B.; Savaris, R.; Lessey, B.A. Medical or surgical treatment before embryo transfer improves outcomes in women with abnormal endometrial BCL6 expression. *J. Assist. Reprod. Genet.* **2019**, *36*, 483–490. [CrossRef]
21. Gong, Q.; Zhu, Y.; Pang, N.; Ai, H.; Gong, X.; La, X.; Ding, J. Increased levels of CCR7(lo)PD-1(hi) CXCR5+ CD4+ T cells, and associated factors Bcl-6, CXCR5, IL-21 and IL-6 contribute to repeated implantation failure. *Exp. Ther. Med.* **2017**, *14*, 5931–5941. [CrossRef] [PubMed]
22. Almquist, L.D.; Likes, C.E.; Stone, B.; Brown, K.R.; Savaris, R.; Forstein, D.A.; Miller, P.B.; Lessey, B.A. Endometrial BCL6 testing for the prediction of in vitro fertilization outcomes: A cohort study. *Fertil. Steril.* **2017**, *108*, 1063–1069. [CrossRef] [PubMed]
23. Moustafa, S.; Young, S. Diagnostic and therapeutic options in recurrent implantation failure. *F1000Res* **2020**, *9*, 208. [CrossRef]
24. Shaffer, A.L.; Yu, X.; He, Y.; Boldrick, J.; Chan, E.P.; Staudt, L.M. BCL-6 represses genes that function in lymphocyte differentiation, inflammation, and cell cycle control. *Immunity* **2000**, *13*, 199–212. [CrossRef] [PubMed]
25. Lee, M.S.; Inoue, T.; Ise, W.; Matsuo-Dapaah, J.; Wing, J.B.; Temizoz, B.; Kobiyama, K.; Hayashi, T.; Patil, A.; Sakaguchi, S.; et al. B cell-intrinsic TBK1 is essential for germinal center formation during infection and vaccination in mice. *J. Exp. Med.* **2021**, *219*, e20211336. [CrossRef]
26. Choi, J.; Crotty, S. Bcl6-Mediated Transcriptional Regulation of Follicular Helper T cells (TFH). *Trends Immunol.* **2021**, *42*, 336–349. [CrossRef]
27. Chen, J.L.; Yang, J.M.; Huang, Y.Z.; Li, Y. Clinical observation of lymphocyte active immunotherapy in 380 patients with unexplained recurrent spontaneous abortion. *Int. Immunopharmacol.* **2016**, *40*, 347–350. [CrossRef]
28. McQueen, D.B.; Perfetto, C.O.; Hazard, F.K.; Lathi, R.B. Pregnancy outcomes in women with chronic endometritis and recurrent pregnancy loss. *Int. Immunopharmacol.* **2016**, *40*, 347–350. [CrossRef]
29. Drury, J.A.; Tang, A.W.; Turner, M.A.; Quenby, S. A rapid, reliable method for uNK cell density estimation. *J. Reprod. Immunol.* **2013**, *97*, 183–185. [CrossRef]
30. Hallager, T.; Saxtorph, M.H.; Eriksen, J.O.; Hviid, T.V.; Macklon, N.S.; Larsen, L.G. Conventional microscopy versus digital image analysis for histopathologic evaluation of immune cells in the endometrium. *J. Reprod. Immunol.* **2021**, *145*, 103294. [CrossRef]
31. Ekemen, S.; Yapicier, O.; Boler, H.D.; Ince, U. An extremely rare case of back and hip pain due to the metastasis of late recurrent myxopapillary ependymoma to the inguinal lymph node. *J. Pathol. Transl. Med.* **2018**, *52*, 67–70. [CrossRef]
32. Herlihy, N.S.; Klimczak, A.M.; Titus, S.; Scott, C.; Hanson, B.M.; Kim, J.K.; Seli, E.; Scott, R.T. The role of endometrial staining for CD138 as a marker of chronic endometritis in predicting live birth. *J. Assist. Reprod. Genet.* **2022**, *39*, 473–479. [CrossRef]

33. Meyerholz, D.K.; Beck, A.P. Principles and approaches for reproducible scoring of tissue stains in research. *Lab. Investig.* **2018**, *98*, 844–855. [CrossRef] [PubMed]
34. Canberk, S.; Behzatoglu, K.; Caliskan, C.K.; Gelmez, S.; Kayhan, K.C.; Aydemir, S.F.; Akbas, M.; Yıldız, I.; Veiga, R.; Alrefae, N.; et al. The Role of Telecytology in the Primary Diagnosis of Thyroid Fine-Needle Aspiration Specimens. *Acta Cytol.* **2019**, *64*, 323–331. [CrossRef] [PubMed]
35. Coulam, C.B. Intralipid treatment for women with reproductive failures. *Am. J. Reprod. Immunol.* **2020**, *85*, e13290. [CrossRef] [PubMed]
36. Liu, Y.; Chen, X.; Huang, J.; Wang, C.-C.; Yu, M.-Y.; Laird, S.; Li, T.-C. Comparison of the prevalence of chronic endometritis as determined by means of different diagnostic methods in women with and without reproductive failure. *Fertil. Steril.* **2018**, *109*, 832–839. [CrossRef] [PubMed]
37. Seshadri, S.; Sunkara, S.K. Natural killer cells in female infertility and recurrent miscarriage: A systematic review and meta-analysis. *Hum. Reprod. Updat.* **2013**, *20*, 429–438. [CrossRef] [PubMed]
38. Quenby, S.; Kalumbi, C.; Bates, M.; Farquharson, R.; Vince, G. Prednisolone reduces preconceptual endometrial natural killer cells in women with recurrent miscarriage. *Fertil. Steril.* **2005**, *84*, 980–984. [CrossRef]
39. Niazi, M.K.K.; Parwani, A.V.; Gurcan, M.N. Digital pathology and artificial intelligence. *Lancet Oncol.* **2019**, *20*, e253–e261. [CrossRef]

Disclaimer/Publisher's Note: The statements, opinions and data contained in all publications are solely those of the individual author(s) and contributor(s) and not of MDPI and/or the editor(s). MDPI and/or the editor(s) disclaim responsibility for any injury to people or property resulting from any ideas, methods, instructions or products referred to in the content.

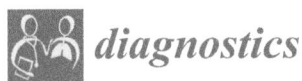

Article

Gestational Diabetes—Placental Expression of Human Equilibrative Nucleoside Transporter 1 (hENT1): Is Delayed Villous Maturation an Adaptive Pattern?

Cinzia Giacometti [1,*], Kathrin Ludwig [2], Monica Guidi [3], Elvira Colantuono [4], Anna Coracina [5], Marcello Rigano [4], Mauro Cassaro [1] and Alessandro Ambrosi [6]

1 Pathology Unit, Department of Diagnostic Services, ULSS 6 "Euganea", 35131 Padova, Italy; mauro.cassaro@aulss6.veneto.it
2 Pathology Unit, Department of Medicine, University of Padova, 35128 Padova, Italy; kathrin.ludwig@aopd.veneto.it
3 Gynecology & Obstretics Unit, Department of Women's Health, Cittadella Hospital, ULSS 6 "Euganea", 35013 Padova, Italy; monica.guidi@aulss6.veneto.it
4 Gynecology & Obstretics Unit, Department of Women's Health, Camposampiero Hospital, ULSS 6 "Euganea", 35012 Padova, Italy; elvira.colantuono@aulss6.veneto.it (E.C.); marcello.rigano@aulss6.veneto.it (M.R.)
5 Diabetology Unit, Department of Medicine, Camposampiero Hospital, ULSS 6 "Euganea", 35012 Padova, Italy; anna.coracina@aulss6.veneto.it
6 School of Medicine, Vita-Salute San Raffaele University, 20132 Milano, Italy; ambrosi.alessandro@hsr.it
* Correspondence: cinzia.giacometti@aulss6.veneto.it

Citation: Giacometti, C.; Ludwig, K.; Guidi, M.; Colantuono, E.; Coracina, A.; Rigano, M.; Cassaro, M.; Ambrosi, A. Gestational Diabetes—Placental Expression of Human Equilibrative Nucleoside Transporter 1 (hENT1): Is Delayed Villous Maturation an Adaptive Pattern? *Diagnostics* **2023**, *13*, 2034. https://doi.org/10.3390/diagnostics13122034

Academic Editor: Valerio Gaetano Vellone

Received: 5 June 2023
Revised: 9 June 2023
Accepted: 10 June 2023
Published: 12 June 2023

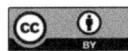

Copyright: © 2023 by the authors. Licensee MDPI, Basel, Switzerland. This article is an open access article distributed under the terms and conditions of the Creative Commons Attribution (CC BY) license (https://creativecommons.org/licenses/by/4.0/).

Abstract: Gestational diabetes mellitus (GDM) is a metabolic disease that can affect placental villous maturation and villous vascularity. The main effects of GDM on placental growth are a delay of villous maturation (DVM) and decreased formation of vasculo-syncytial membranes (VSM). Human equilibrative nucleoside transporter-1 (hENT1) is an adenosine transporter expressed in the human umbilical vein endothelial cells (HUVEC) and human placental microvascular endothelium cells (hPMEC). Its role is crucial in maintaining physiological fetal adenosine levels during pregnancy, and its reduction has been described in GDM. Twenty-four placentas from pregnancies with a confirmed diagnosis of GDMd and twenty-four matched non-GDM placentas (controls) were retrospectively analyzed to investigate the immunohistochemical expression of hENT1 in HUVEC and hPMEC. The study included the quantitative evaluation of VSM/mm^2 in placental tissue and the immunohistochemical quantitative evaluation of Ki-67, PHH3, and p57 in villous trophoblast. hENT1 expression was higher in all the vascular districts of the control cases compared to the GDMd placentas ($p < 0.0001$). The VSM/mm^2 were lower in the GDMd cases, while the Ki-67, PHH3, and p57 were higher when compared to the control cases. To our knowledge, this is the first report of hENT1 expression in the human placentas of GDM patients. The absence/low expression of hENT1 in all the GDMd patients may indicate a potential role in microvascular adaptive mechanisms. The trophoblasts' proliferative/antiapoptotic pattern (high Ki-67, high PHH3, and high p57 count) may explain the statistically significant lower number of VSM/mm^2 found in the GDMd cases.

Keywords: gestational diabetes; placenta; hENT1; vasculo-syncytial membrane; Ki-67; p57

1. Introduction

Gestational diabetes mellitus (GDM) is a disease defined by its onset or first recognition during pregnancy and is characterized by glucose intolerance, leading to maternal hyperglycemia. Its incidence accounts for 15% of pregnancies in developed and developing countries [1]. Although GDM resolves after birth, it is associated with changes during prenatal life, perinatal alterations (e.g., macrosomia, insulin resistance, and higher systolic blood pressure), and diseases in adulthood (e.g., diabetes, obesity, dyslipidemia, hypertension, and metabolic syndrome) [2–6].

One pathophysiological consequence of GMD is altered vascular function, defined as the altered capacity of the endothelium to take up and metabolize the cationic amino acid L-arginine, the substrate for NO synthesis via NO synthases (NOS) [7,8]. Since the placenta lacks innervation, the physiological vascular placental function is maintained by locally released vasoactive molecules from the endothelium, such as the gas nitric oxide (NO) or the endogenous nucleoside adenosine [9]. Adenosine is a vasodilator in most vascular beds, including the human placenta. The main biological effects of adenosine are to maintain the homeostatic equilibrium and act as a key stimulator of angiogenesis. The latter results in increased L-arginine transport-dependent NO synthesis via the endothelial NO synthase. Thus, a functional link between adenosine and the endothelial L-arginine/NO pathway (ALANO pathway) has been proposed [9]. Human equilibrative nucleoside transporter-1 (hENT1) is an adenosine transporter expressed in human umbilical vein endothelial cells (HUVEC) and human placenta microvascular endothelium cells (hPMEC) [10,11]. In HUVEC, adenosine transport is mainly mediated by hENT1. HUVEC and hPMEC are known to be metabolically crucial in maintaining normal adenosine extracellular levels by efficient uptake of this nucleoside [12], thus modulating its broad biological effects. Differential expression of adenosine receptor subtypes is a factor known to contribute to the functional heterogeneity of human placental macro- and microvascular endothelium. Its role is crucial in maintaining physiological fetal adenosine levels in utero, and its reduction has been described in GDM pregnancies in cultured cells derived from GDM placentas and umbilical cords. This phenomenon is associated with a lower capacity of adenosine transport via human equilibrative nucleoside transporters (hENTs) by HUVEC and hPMEC in GDM [12]. The histological hallmark of the effects of GDM on placental maturation is the so-called delay of villous maturation (DVM), which also encompasses the decreased formation of vasculo-syncytial membranes, the presence of multiple centrally located capillaries and a variable extent of chorangiosis [13,14]. Placental villous maturation reaches the highest point in the 3rd trimester, with an abundance of terminal villi, defined by small-caliber vessels (40–100 μm), minimal stroma, and abundant vasculo-syncytial membrane (VSM) formation [15]. The VSM is the structure that must allow and facilitate the optimal gas exchange between the maternal blood lakes and the fetal bloodstream through the placental villi. The VSM derives from the "fusion" of fetal capillary walls, which are peripherally located, in strict proximity to the trophoblast basement membrane and an ultra-thin layer of trophoblast cytoplasm. At term, terminal villi account for 40–50% of the placental volume and 60% of the cross-sectional area [16]. Delayed villous maturation (DVM) is an entity by which the maturation of the terminal placental villi is abnormal, and it takes place to a lesser extent for gestational age [17]. The villi are usually large and enlarged, with a higher number of stromal cells and edematous stroma. Many capillaries are not peripherally located on higher-power magnification, resulting in a decrease in VSM formation. The trophoblast surrounding the villi appears thickened and hypercellular [18]. The placentas of GDM women are usually larger, thicker, and heavier compared to those of women with normal pregnancies. Even if the exact mechanisms accounting for the increased placental mass remain mainly unclear, some suggestions of alterations in trophoblast cells' proliferation, differentiation, and cell death have been proposed. Some authors described an increase in cellular proliferation markers, detected by proliferative cell nuclear antigen (PCNA) and Ki-67, in the various villous cell types: cytotrophoblasts, syncytiotrophoblasts, stromal cells, and endothelial cells [19]. Although these changes may contribute to the well-known increased placental size, an alternative hypothesis suggests a possible cause in the dysregulation of trophoblast cell death [20]. Together with Ki-67, another marker of cell proliferation is the phosphorylation of histone H3 at serine10 (H3S10P). This is an important event in the cell cycle progression, starting in the pericentromeric chromatin in the late G2 phase. The process then spreads non-randomly throughout the condensing chromatin during the prophase, persisting throughout the anaphase of the cell cycle. As phosphohistone H3 (PHH3) phosphorylation is typically no longer detectable when mitosis is completed and is not expressed in apoptotic bodies, it is a specific marker of mitotic figures [21]. p57 is a protein of the CIP/KIP family of cyclin-dependent kinase (CDK) inhibitors (CKIs). In human placentas, it is present in the villous cytotrophoblasts, villous stromal cells, amniotic epithelium, invasive cytotrophoblasts, and decidual cells. Due to its role in cell cycle control, p57 is involved in regulating a variety of cellular processes, such as embryogenesis and tissue differentiation, and its regulation is highly complex. p57 has a highly specific profile expression, both spatially and temporally: its peak and widespread distribution are at a maximum during embryogenesis and development. At the same time, it remains restricted to only a few tissues in adult life [22].

This study aimed to investigate the immunohistochemical expression of hENT1 in HUVEC and hPMEC in delivered placentas of GDM patients in dietary treatment (GDMd). The study included the quantitative evaluation of the VSM, Ki-67, PHH3, and p57 and their correlation with hENT1 and fetal, placental, and maternal characteristics.

2. Materials and Methods

This retrospective observational study did not imply any change in therapeutic or diagnostic procedures. Only intact placentas and patients with available clinical data and analysis were considered in the study. Placentas from patients with a GDMd diagnosis and no other co-morbidities were consecutively collected in the ULSS 6 Community Hospitals of Camposampiero and Cittadella (Padua, Italy) from April to July 2018. A diagnosis of GDM was achieved in the presence of at least one glycemic level above the normal in the two-hour test with 75 g syrup glucose solution: equal to or higher than 92 mg/dL (5.11 mmol/L) immediately after (time 0) and/or equal to or higher than 180 mg/dL (10 mmol/L) after 60 min and/or equal to or higher than 153 mg/dL (8.5 mmol/L) after 120 min [1]. Control cases, with normal glucose tolerance tests during pregnancy, were collected from consecutive deliveries in the same period. All the delivered placentas were formalin-fixed and paraffine-embedded (FFPE) after 2–4 days of 4% buffered formalin fixation. Placental sampling was conducted according to the Amsterdam protocol [17], modified as follows: A total of six samples were collected from every placenta: one sample of membranes (membrane roll) and umbilical cord (proximal, intermediate, and distal, near to cord insertion), one sample including cord insertion, three samples of placental parenchyma (two center-parenchymal, one of the most and one of the least normal area, and one para-central sample. All the diagnoses were rendered according to the Amsterdam protocol, as follows: delayed villous maturation (DVM), maternal vascular malperfusion (MVM), chorioamnionitis, villitis of unknown etiology (VUE), or a combination of two (or more) diagnoses (MVM + DVM, MVM + chorioamnionitis, etc.). The mid-portion of the placental parenchyma was assessed in 1 section from each placenta. Four consecutive high-power fields (about 1 mm^2; field diameter 0.62 mm; field area 0.302 mm^2) were evaluated, and the VSM were counted in all the terminal villi present in each field [16]. The same slide used for the VSM evaluation was incubated with p57 (mouse monoclonal antibody, 5 mL dispenser, pre-diluted, ~1.3 µg/mL, Roche Diagnostics), Ki-67 (clone 30-9, rabbit monoclonal antibody, 5 mL dispenser, pre-diluted, ~2 µg/mL, Roche Diagnostics), and PHH3 (rabbit polyclonal antibody, 5 mL dispenser, pre-diluted, ~1.3 µg/mL, Cell Marque, Sigma Aldrich). Ki-67 and p57 were scored by counting the percentage of positive nuclei on 200 villous syncytiotrophoblast cells; PHH3 immunohistochemistry was scored by counting the positive nuclei/mm^2 (as reported above) in villous syncytiotrophoblast cells. Umbilical cord and placental parenchyma samples from the GDMd cases and non-GDM controls were incubated with hENT-1 antibody (clone sp120, rabbit monoclonal antibody, pre-diluted, ~0.44 µg/mL, Roche Diagnostics); incubation without the primary antibody served as a negative control. According to the manufacturer's instructions, the normal pancreas served as a positive control. As hENT1 immunohistochemical expression is not reported in the literature applied to the human placenta, its expression was quantitatively evaluated in the HUVEC and hPMEC using the proportion of positive cells and multiplying the percentage of cells demonstrating each intensity and adding the results, as for the $H-score = \sum_{i=0}^{3} i \cdot p_i$ described for the quantification of estrogen and progesterone receptor expression in the breast, where i is the intensity score (scored from 0, absent, to 3, strong, intense reaction) and p_i is the corresponding percentage of the cell [23]. A score between 0 and 300 was achieved for each case and in each vascular district (HUVEC and hPMEC). The syncytiotrophoblast cells' basement membranes served as the positive internal control.

2.1. Statistical Methods

2.1.1. Pre-Processing

After a preliminary check, we used the propensity score to select samples of matching subjects to reduce the possible risk of bias due to confounding variables. We used logistic regression to estimate the propensity scores considering the following covariates: BMI and age at delivery, fetal/placental weight ratio (F/P), and placental/fetal weight ratio (P/F). We matched (1:1) the cases and controls using the optimal matching approach, which keeps the sum of the absolute pairwise distances in the matched sample as small as possible, without replacement. We assessed the balance in the distribution of the covariates before and after matching using the standardized mean difference and variance ratio (an absolute standardized mean difference of <0.2 after matching was considered to indicate a good balance) and checked the test power. The following analyses were applied to the matched samples.

2.1.2. Analysis

The observed numeric values were summarized by the mean and standard deviation (SD), and the categorical values were summarized by frequencies and percentages. To allow an easier comparison with the literature, the complete descriptive statistics are reported in the Supplementary Material. The correlation between the numeric variables was computed by means of Spearman's correlation coefficient, ρ. The difference in the means between the cases and controls was assessed by means of Welch's t-type test. The dependencies between the categorical variables were assessed with Fisher's test or the Chi-squared test.

To find subgroups of patients, we performed an unsupervised hierarchical cluster analysis based on the following: maternal variables (diastolic arterial pressure, systolic arterial pressure, BMI at delivery), fetal variables (APGAR score al 5', fetal weight, gestational weeks), placental variables (umbilical cord index—UCI—defined as the number of umbilical vein coils/cm, placental diameters—maximum and minimum, placental weight, umbilical cord diameters—maximum and minimum, placental thickness—maximum and minimum), immunohistochemical variables (expression of p57, proliferation index scored by Ki-67, expression of hENT1 in PMEC, expression of hENT1 in HUVEC), and morphological variables (number of vasculo-syncytial membranes/mm^2, VSM/mm^2). The hierarchical clustering was based on Ward's criterion with the Euclidean distance for the patients and the pairwise correlational distance $(1 - |\rho|)$ for the variables. We graphically represented the results as heatmaps with dendrograms obtained from both complete hierarchical clustering results. We applied a least absolute shrinkage and selection operator (LASSO) to a logistic regression model considering all the variables included in the cluster analyses to identify a minimum set of the most informative variables. The variables with a nonzero coefficient in the LASSO logistic model were selected as a set of potential predictors. Finally, we checked the capability to classify the GDMd versus non-GDM cases of the selected variables by an optimism-adjusted Sommer's D index based on bootstrap (B = 20,000) and the associated classification accuracy. To further graphically inspect the capability of the selected variables to identify the two groups of patients, we plotted the first two dimensions of the Principal Component Analysis (PCA), along with the elliptic convex hull of the cases and controls. Exact p-values were computed by means of permutation methods to avoid any distributional approximation, and the significance level was set at $\alpha = 0.05$. All the statistical analyses were performed with R (version 4.2.1).

3. Results

A total number of 81 consecutive placentas were submitted to the Pathology Laboratory between April and July 2018, according to the guidelines [24]. Of these, two were excluded because of incomplete clinical or laboratory data and three were excluded due to fragmentation during delivery (manual removal of the afterbirth). All the remaining placentas (n = 76) fulfilled the inclusion/exclusion criteria: 28 placentas from diagnosed GDMd mothers (cases) and 48 placentas associated with non-GDM diagnoses (controls). After 1:1 propensity score matching, 24 GDM cases were matched with 24 non-GDM controls (6 intra-uterine growth restrictions, 6 cases of fetal distress during labor, 3 cases suspicious for placenta accreta, 2 placentas with small for gestational age fetuses, 2 cases of premature rupture of membranes, 1 pre-term delivery, 1 maternal fever during labor, 1 oligohydramnios, 1 case of hepatogestosis, 1 placenta previa). The resulting sample size allowed a test power of $1 - \beta = 0.95$ with respect to Cohen's effect size $d = 0.8$ and a significance level $\alpha = 0.05$.

The patient, newborn, and delivery characteristics are summarized in Table 1.

Table 1. Clinical characteristics of pregnant women, newborns, and deliveries.

Variable	GDMd (Mean ± SD)	Non-GDM (Mean ± SD)	
Mothers			p
Age (yrs)	34.62 ± 4.28	33.67 ± 4.69	0.48
BMI (kg/m^2)			
Pre-pregnancy	24.19 ± 4.85	23.98 ± 4.23	0.87
At term	27.77 ± 4.32	28.145 ± 4.55	0.78
Systolic blood pressure (mmHg)	118.75 ± 11.07	123.75 ± 18.14	0.25
Diastolic blood pressure (mmHg)	73.08 ± 9.32	74.67 ± 10.98	0.60
OGTT (mg/dL)		Not performed	
Basal glycemia	86.04 ± 9.34	-	
1-h glycemia after glucose load	162.08 ± 29.03	-	
2-h glycemia after glucose load	153.87 ± 25.98	-	
Newborns			
Sex (female/male)	12/12	13/11	
Gestational age (weeks)	39.05 ± 1.11	37.95 ± 2.49	0.056
Birth weight (grams)	3248.54 ± 481.66	2626.12 ± 568.67	0.0002
Placenta/fetus ratio	0.14 ± 0.02	0.14 ± 0.02	0.87
APGAR score (5 min)	9.83 ± 0.38	9.21 ± 0.97	0.007
Deliveries			
Type of delivery			
Vaginal, spontaneous, n (%)	10/24 (41.67%)	11/24 (45.83%)	
Vaginal, induced, n (%)	13/24 (54.17%)	1/24 (4.16%)	
Caesarian, n (%)	1/24 (4.16%)	10/24 (41.67%)	
Operative, n (%)	0/24 (0%)	2/24 (8.34%)	

According to the Amsterdam protocol, the histological diagnoses of GDMd cases consisted of DVM in 20 cases (83.3%) and DVM with focal features of MVM in 4 cases (16.7%). Among the control cases, 12 cases (50%) were diagnosed as MVM with focal features of DVM, 8 cases (33.3%) as MVM, 2 cases (8.3%) as normal placenta with infections (chorioamnionitis), 1 case (4.2%) as VUE, and 1 case (4.2%) as normal. As expected, the GDMd placentas were heavier (477.54 ± 75.96 g versus 394.91 ± 120.96 g, $p = 0.0007$) and the GDMd fetal weight was higher (3248.54 ± 501.07 versus 2626.12 ± 568.66 g, $p < 0.0001$) than in the non-GDM cases. There was no statistical difference between the two groups with regard to the BMI at term and ΔBMI. The mean expression of hENT1 in the control cases versus the GDMd placentas was 159.17 ± 54.76 versus 10 ± 23.03 in the hPMEC ($p < 0.0001$) and 194.17 ± 66.52 versus 11.25 ± 21.93 in the HUVEC ($p < 0.0001$) (Figure 1).

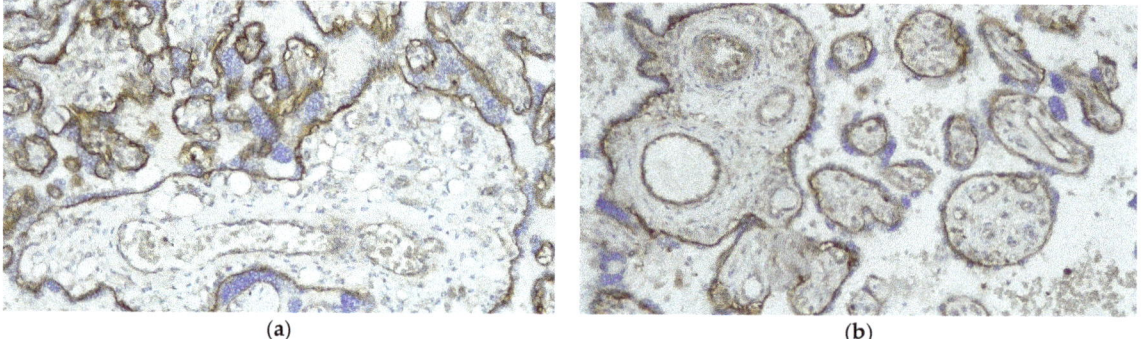

Figure 1. Placental tissue, hENT1 expression. The basement membrane of the villous trophoblast served as a positive internal control. (**a**) GDMd case, hENT 1 expression, score 0 in hPMEC (original magnification 20×); large, "edematous" terminal villi, with centrally located vessels and a continuous layer of syncytiotrophoblasts, which decorates the villi circumferentially. The centrally located vessels are negative for hENT1. VSMs are minimally formed. (**b**) non-GDM case, MVM, hENT 1 expression, score 250 in hPMEC (original magnification 20×). In MVM, the terminal villi are often smaller than usual, often with a "pencil-like" shape (so-called accelerated maturation). Syncytial knots are prominent. The syncytiotrophoblast layer is mainly polarized. All the vessels are positive for hENT1.

The Ki-67, PHH3, and p57 counts were significantly higher in the GDMd group when compared to the controls (Ki-67 count 19.95 ± 2.83 versus 7.5 ± 2.37, $p < 0.0001$; PHH3 count 3.79 ± 2.26 versus 0.96 ± 0.80, $p < 0.0001$; p57 count 20.87 ± 4.72 vs 8.45 ± 2.84, $p < 0.0001$). This "proliferative"/antiapoptotic pattern (high Ki-67, PHH3, and p57 counts) seems to sustain the statistically significantly lower number of VSM/mm^2 found in the GDMd cases compared to the controls (3.67 ± 2.96 versus 20.04 ± 8.77; $p < 0.0001$) (Figure 2).

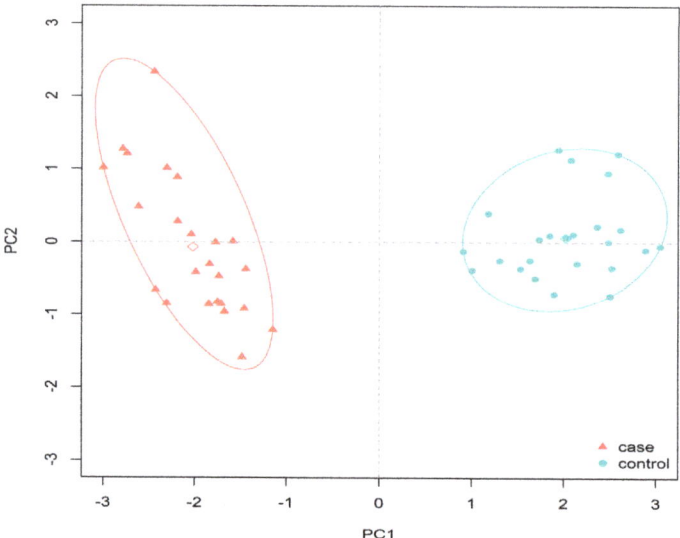

Figure 2. Plot of the first two Principal Components after LASSO feature selection, with elliptic convex hull for cases (GDMd) and controls (non-GDM) patients. The first two components account for 84.21% of the total variability. Empty diamonds represent the mean values (First Principal Component loadings: hENT1 HUVEC = 0.429, hENT1 hPMEC = 0.421, VSM = 0.373, Ki-67 = −0.444, PHH3 = −0.345, p57 = −0.428).

Bootstrap-based resampling gave an optimism-corrected Sommer's D index of 1 and a mean accuracy equal to 100%. However, we underline that these results should be taken carefully, given the final sample size. The main results are summarized in Table 2 and Figure 3.

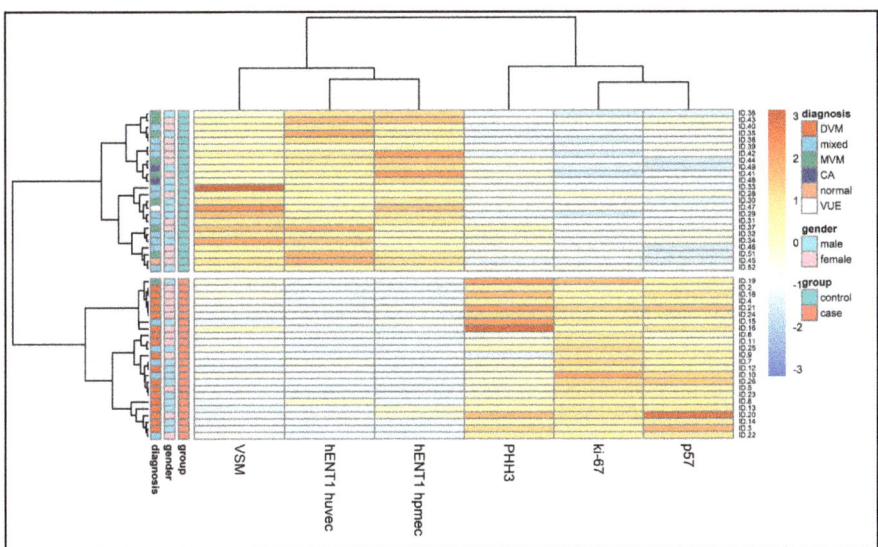

Figure 3. Heatmap of 24 GDMd patients matched with 24 non-GDM patients. After a LASSO-based selection, only six features were retained as informative. Hierarchical clustering was based on Euclidean distance for patients and pairwise correlational distance $(1 - |\rho|)$ for features.

Table 2. Morphological characteristics of placentas and immunohistochemical findings.

Variable	GDMd (Mean ± SD)	Non-GDM (Mean ± SD)	p
Morphological findings			
Weight (grams)	477.54 ± 75.96	394.91 ± 120.96	0.007
Diameter (cm)			
Maximum	17.29 ± 1.89	16.26 ± 1.86	0.07
Minimum	15.21 ± 1.61	14.10 ± 2.02	0.04
Thickness (cm)			
Maximum	3.48 ± 0.59	3.41 ± 0.82	0.76
Minimum	1.73 ± 0.80	1.49 ± 0.78	0.30
Cord length (cm)	27.08 ± 7.38	30.85 ± 11.97	0.10
Umbilical Cord Index (UCI, number of umbilical veins twists/cm)	0.32 ± 0.12	0.32 ± 0.22	0.94
Histological diagnosis	**GDMd**	**Non-GDM**	
Number of cases, %	DVM 20 (83.3%)	MVM 12 (50%)	
	DVM + MVM 4 (16.7%)	MVM + DVM 8 (33%)	
		CA 2 (8.3%)	
		VUE 1 (4.2%)	
		Normal 1 (4.2%)	

Table 2. *Cont.*

Immunohistochemical and morphological study	GDMd (mean ± SD)	Non-GDM (mean ± SD)	p
hENT1 HUVEC	11.25 ± 21.93	194.17 ± 66.52	<0.0001
hENT1 hPMEC	10.00 ± 23.03	159.17 ± 54.76	<0.0001
Ki-67	19.96 ± 2.83	7.50 ± 2.37	<0.0001
PHH3	3.79 ± 2.26	0.96 ± 0.80	<0.0001
p57	20.87 ± 4.72	8.45 ± 2.84	<0.0001
VSM	3.67 ± 2.96	20.04 ± 8.77	<0.0001

4. Discussion

The screening strategies for GDM used across Europe still bear many differences between countries. By applying selective screening according to European guidelines, approximately 50% of pregnant women would need to be subjected to a glucose tolerance test. The application of Dutch guidelines permits the reduction of the percentage of undiagnosed cases ("only" 33%) [25]. Insulin therapy could be clinically considered useful to restore normal maternal and fetal glycemia when dietary therapy is insufficient; however, its usefulness in avoiding endothelial dysfunction is still unclear [26]. This could be due, as previously demonstrated in in vitro models, to the incapacity of insulin therapy per se to restore fully normal vascular functionality in GDM placenta micro-macrovasculature [27]. Insulin stimulates fetal aerobic glucose metabolism and will increase the fetus's oxygen demand. If adequate supply is not available due to reduced oxygen delivery (to the intervillous space because of the higher oxygen affinity of glycated hemoglobin, thickening of the placental basement membrane, and reduced uteroplacental or fetoplacental blood flow), fetal hypoxemia will ensue, despite therapy. Maternal diabetes has several effects on the human placenta. Characteristically, the placenta in GDM, as we also demonstrated in the present study, is heavier and thicker, with an enlarged surface area of exchange both on the maternal (syncytiotrophoblast) and fetal (endothelium) side. It may appear paradoxical that in a situation of maternal nutritional oversupply, the placenta increases its weight, thickness, and surface, thus potentially contributing to enhanced maternal-fetal transport. This kind of adaptation reflects both the crucial importance of guaranteeing an adequate oxygen supply to the fetus and the effect of excess growth factors (such as insulin), which drives some of the placental changes, even if they result in adverse side effects. If morphology may give a clue about the pathogenesis of structural placenta abnormalities, the molecular substrate may provide a possible answer, as clinical manifestations of GDM seem to rely on fetoplacental endothelial dysfunction [7]. Different mechanisms leading to vascular alterations present in GDM have been investigated. Among these, the reduced adenosine uptake due to reduced hENT1 transport capacity has been widely investigated [28,29]. Adenosine is an endogenous purine nucleoside formed in both intra- and extracellular spaces. The production of extracellular adenosine originates from the dephosphorylation of extracellular adenosine monophosphate via the nucleotidases displayed in the plasma membrane of endothelial cells [30], including HUVEC [31]. Adenosine plays many different roles in vascular tissues, such as the regulation of vascular tone and blood flow [10]. The abnormally elevated extracellular adenosine concentration described in the culture medium of HUVEC may lead to the activation of adenosine receptors, which could repress adenosine transport via hENT1 in hPMEC [27]. These could be crucial mechanisms in the maintenance of physiological extracellular adenosine levels both in the micro-and macro-circulation of the human placenta in GDM [32]. The efficiency in adenosine uptake has been reported to be altered in isolated HUVEC from GDMd patients, so it was postulated that a reduction in hENT1 likely occurred in the endothelial cells [9]. Endothelial dysfunction is a crucial aspect of GDM. In 2013, Pardo et al. [33] reviewed the role of adenosine and its receptors in GDM. In their exhaustive review, they highlighted the existing link between nitric oxide (NO) and the adenosine pathway in the so-called ALANO pathway [7]. According to this hypothesis, HUVEC and hPMEC from GDM patients result in higher levels of NO, a functional severance between NO synthase and L-arginine uptake, increased levels of adenosine, and reduced expression of hENT1 [33–35]. In our study, we investigated the presence of the immunohistochemical expression of hENT1 in different vascular districts in GDMd placentas and non-GDM placentas. We demonstrated that hENT1 membrane expression is largely diminished or absent in GDMd placentas, while it remains largely unaltered in all other cases. This phenomenon has been observed both in HUVEC and hPMEC, compared to control cases with normal basal glycemia. In non-GDMd cases, hENT1 expression was moderate to strong and diffusely present in all the vascular districts investigated; for this reason, the absence/reduction of hENT1 expression is likely to identify potential GDMd placentas, even in the absence of clinically/serological proven GDM. One of the theses postulated in this paper is that the peculiar morphological aspect of placental tissue (larger, "edematous", hypervascularized, and immature villi) in GDM patients (the so-called DVM) [17] is the expression of an adaptive mechanism apt to reduce fetal exposure to the highly oxidative environment caused by hyperglycemia and hyperinsulinism rather than a true immatureness of the villous population. Hyperglycemia and hyperinsulinemia of diabetic pregnancies may be one of several mechanisms by which DVM occurs, but in a previous study, no differences between glycosylated hemoglobin or fructosamine values in pregestational diabetic patients with or without DVM were identified [36]. Various etiologies for the pathogenesis of DVM have been suggested, including increased levels of placental growth factors, as seen in diabetes and maternal obesity [37]. At the microscopic level, the specific histological feature of GDM is DVM, with rates in diabetic placentas ranging from 81% [38] to 16.6% [18]. We assume that DVM could be a misnomer, as the villi in GDM patients are not truly immature, even if they display a morphology similar to the villi from the 33rd to 34th weeks of gestation. In our opinion, the lack of formation of the VSM might be a protective mechanism in GDM placentas rather than an unwanted side effect of hyperglycemia and hyperinsulinemia. The inadequate number of VSM in the terminal villi of GDM placentas, probably due to the higher proliferation of villous syncytiotrophoblasts (higher Ki-67 value and mitosis number), creates a physical barrier between the intervillous maternal blood and fetal villous capillaries, thickening the virtual space of the VSM by the proliferation of trophoblastic cells. This barrier could be useful in reducing the maternal oversupply to the fetus. In contrast to other previous work [19] we found an increase in p57 expression in syncytiotrophoblast cells. We hypothesized that p57 expression in GDMd placentas is modulated by the oxidative environment: the oxidative stress would act as an antiapoptotic stimulus rather than a proapoptotic one [22], leading to the persistence of "immature", circumferential syncytiotrophoblasts, which does not involve creating the normal, polarized, syncytial knot usually seen in normal terminal villi. In this way, the syncytiotrophoblast cytoplasm helps create a physical barrier to the formation of the VSM.

5. Conclusions

The empirical results reported herein should be considered in light of some limitations.

The retrospective nature of the study did not allow for the collection of all the precise potential data about the mother's health and pregnancy. This problem could be easily encompassed by the prospective enrollment of patients and via the use of adequate surveys to explore dietary and lifestyle habits apt to produce effects on pregnancies. We could not enroll insulin-treated patients as there are many different therapeutic schemes and they were not always clearly retrievable by existing databases.

We also acknowledge that the sample size is limited due to limited resources and that the control group is heterogeneous concerning the placental pathology. The latter is due to the adherence to the guidelines regarding the referral of the placentas to the Pathology Laboratory, so placentas delivered from normal pregnancies are not available. At any rate, the cases and controls were matched by the propensity scores. The study was further limited by the absence of previous research studies on this specific topic. Prior research relevant to our thesis is scarce and exquisitely experimental, based on cell cultures isolated from placental tissue; for these reasons, we had to develop a completely new approach, based on placental tissue and immunohistochemistry.

Our work seems to corroborate, not regarding the cultured cells but the placental tissue, the hypothesis that the absence/low expression of hENT1 in endothelial cells in all GDMd placentas may indicate a potential role in microvascular adaptive mechanisms. As the placental microenvironment is extremely complex, many different pathways and metabolic mechanisms likely rely on the alterations found both at cellular and phenotypic levels in GDM. We described a "proliferative"/antiapoptotic pattern (high Ki-67, PHH3, and p57 counts) in the GDMd placentas, which seems to sustain the statistically significant lower number of VSM/mm^2 found in the GDMd cases when compared to the controls. The combination of the peculiar GDM parameters (absence of hENT1, lower VSM count, high MIB1, PHH3, and p57) could discriminate between GDM (irrespective of morphological features) and non-GDM placentas. Future studies should investigate the expression of hENT1 in non-clinically evident GDM and insulin-treated GDM patients.

Supplementary Materials: The following supporting information can be downloaded at: https://www.mdpi.com/article/10.3390/diagnostics13122034/s1.

Author Contributions: C.G. performed the study concept and the design, development of the methodology and the writing, review, and revision of the paper; K.L. and A.A. performed the development of the methodology and the writing, review, and revision of the paper. A.A. performed the analysis and interpretation of the data and the statistical analysis. M.G., A.C., E.C., M.R. and M.C. provided the acquisition of the data. All authors have read and agreed to the published version of the manuscript.

Funding: This research received no external funding.

Institutional Review Board Statement: The study was conducted in accordance with the Declaration of Helsinki. The ethical review and approval were waived for this study because this retrospective observational study did not imply any change in the therapeutic or diagnostic routinary procedure.

Informed Consent Statement: Patient consent was waived because this retrospective observational study did not imply any change in the therapeutic or diagnostic routinary procedure.

Data Availability Statement: The data are available upon request due to restrictions (privacy). The data presented in this study are available upon request from the corresponding author.

Acknowledgments: We would like to thank Luciana Poletto, Patrizia Peruffo, Sara Ghiretti, and Lucetta Vidotto for their technical support and the midwives Donatella De Palma, Alessandra Presa, Anna Gazzola Martini, and Veronica Ventre for their help in collecting the cases.

Conflicts of Interest: The authors declare no conflict of interest.

References

1. American Diabetes Association. Diagnosis and classification of diabetes mellitus. *Diabetes Care* **2013**, *36* (Suppl. 1), S67–S74. [CrossRef]
2. Sivaraman, S.C.; Vinnamala, S.; Jenkins, D. Gestational diabetes and future risk of diabetes. *J. Clin. Med. Res.* **2013**, *5*, 92–96. [CrossRef] [PubMed]
3. Buchanan, T.A.; Xiang, A.H.; Page, K.A. Gestational diabetes mellitus: Risks and management during and after pregnancy. *Nat. Rev. Endocrinol.* **2012**, *8*, 639–649. [CrossRef]
4. Metzger, B.E.; Coustan, D.R.; Trimble, E.R. Hyperglycemia and Adverse Pregnancy Outcomes. *Clin. Chem.* **2019**, *65*, 937–938. [CrossRef] [PubMed]
5. Landon, M.B.; Mele, L.; Varner, M.W.; Casey, B.M.; Reddy, U.M.; Wapner, R.J.; Rouse, D.J.; Tita, A.T.N.; Thorp, J.M.; Chien, E.K.; et al. The relationship of maternal glycemia to childhood obesity and metabolic dysfunction. *J. Matern. Fetal Neonatal Med.* **2020**, *33*, 33–41. [CrossRef] [PubMed]
6. Gao, M.; Cao, S.; Li, N.; Liu, J.; Lyu, Y.; Li, J.; Yang, X. Risks of overweight in the offspring of women with gestational diabetes at different developmental stages: A meta-analysis with more than half a million offspring. *Obes. Rev.* **2022**, *23*, e13395. [CrossRef]
7. Leiva, A.; Pardo, F.; Ramirez, M.A.; Farias, M.; Casanello, P.; Sobrevia, L. Fetoplacental vascular endothelial dysfunction as an early phenomenon in the programming of human adult diseases in subjects born from gestational diabetes mellitus or obesity in pregnancy. *Exp. Diabetes Res.* **2011**, *2011*, 349286. [CrossRef] [PubMed]

8. Guzman-Gutierrez, E.; Abarzua, F.; Belmar, C.; Nien, J.K.; Ramirez, M.A.; Arroyo, P.; Salomon, C.; Westermeier, F.; Puebla, C.; Leiva, A.; et al. Functional link between adenosine and insulin: A hypothesis for fetoplacental vascular endothelial dysfunction in gestational diabetes. *Curr. Vasc. Pharmacol.* **2011**, *9*, 750–762. [CrossRef]
9. San Martin, R.; Sobrevia, L. Gestational diabetes and the adenosine/L-arginine/nitric oxide (ALANO) pathway in human umbilical vein endothelium. *Placenta* **2006**, *27*, 1–10. [CrossRef]
10. Baldwin, S.A.; Beal, P.R.; Yao, S.Y.; King, A.E.; Cass, C.E.; Young, J.D. The equilibrative nucleoside transporter family, SLC29. *Pflug. Arch.* **2004**, *447*, 735–743. [CrossRef]
11. Guzman-Gutierrez, E.; Sandoval, C.; Nova, E.; Castillo, J.L.; Vera, J.C.; Lamperti, L.; Krause, B.; Salomon, C.; Sepulveda, C.; Aguayo, C.; et al. Differential expression of functional nucleoside transporters in non-differentiated and differentiated human endothelial progenitor cells. *Placenta* **2010**, *31*, 928–936. [CrossRef]
12. Sobrevia, L.; Abarzua, F.; Nien, J.K.; Salomon, C.; Westermeier, F.; Puebla, C.; Cifuentes, F.; Guzman-Gutierrez, E.; Leiva, A.; Casanello, P. Review: Differential placental macrovascular and microvascular endothelial dysfunction in gestational diabetes. *Placenta* **2011**, *32* (Suppl. 2), S159–S164. [CrossRef]
13. Treacy, A.; Higgins, M.; Kearney, J.M.; McAuliffe, F.; Mooney, E.E. Delayed villous maturation of the placenta: Quantitative assessment in different cohorts. *Pediatr. Dev. Pathol.* **2013**, *16*, 63–66. [CrossRef] [PubMed]
14. Giacometti, C.; Cassaro, M. Clinicopathologic Correlations in Histopathologic Report of Placenta: Can We Do Something More? *Arch. Pathol. Lab. Med.* **2017**, *141*, 184–185. [CrossRef] [PubMed]
15. Saha, S.; Biswas, S.; Mitra, D.; Adhikari, A.; Saha, C. Histologic and morphometric study of human placenta in gestational diabetes mellitus. *Ital. J. Anat. Embryol.* **2014**, *119*, 1–9. [PubMed]
16. Sala, M.A.; Matheus, M. Regional variation of the vasculo-syncytial membranes in the human full-term placenta. *Gegenbaurs Morphol. Jahrb.* **1986**, *132*, 285–289.
17. Khong, T.Y.; Mooney, E.E.; Ariel, I.; Balmus, N.C.; Boyd, T.K.; Brundler, M.A.; Derricott, H.; Evans, M.J.; Faye-Petersen, O.M.; Gillan, J.E.; et al. Sampling and Definitions of Placental Lesions: Amsterdam Placental Workshop Group Consensus Statement. *Arch. Pathol. Lab. Med.* **2016**, *140*, 698–713. [CrossRef] [PubMed]
18. Higgins, M.; McAuliffe, F.M.; Mooney, E.E. Clinical associations with a placental diagnosis of delayed villous maturation: A retrospective study. *Pediatr. Dev. Pathol.* **2011**, *14*, 273–279. [CrossRef] [PubMed]
19. Unek, G.; Ozmen, A.; Mendilcioglu, I.; Simsek, M.; Korgun, E.T. Immunohistochemical distribution of cell cycle proteins p27, p57, cyclin D3, PCNA and Ki67 in normal and diabetic human placentas. *J. Mol. Histol.* **2014**, *45*, 21–34. [CrossRef] [PubMed]
20. Hung, T.H.; Huang, S.Y.; Chen, S.F.; Wu, C.P.; Hsieh, T.T. Decreased placental apoptosis and autophagy in pregnancies complicated by gestational diabetes with large-for-gestational age fetuses. *Placenta* **2020**, *90*, 27–36. [CrossRef]
21. Tetzlaff, M.T.; Curry, J.L.; Ivan, D.; Wang, W.L.; Torres-Cabala, C.A.; Bassett, R.L.; Valencia, K.M.; McLemore, M.S.; Ross, M.I.; Prieto, V.G. Immunodetection of phosphohistone H3 as a surrogate of mitotic figure count and clinical outcome in cutaneous melanoma. *Mod. Pathol.* **2013**, *26*, 1153–1160. [CrossRef]
22. Rossi, M.N.; Antonangeli, F. Cellular Response upon Stress: p57 Contribution to the Final Outcome. *Mediat. Inflamm.* **2015**, *2015*, 259325. [CrossRef]
23. McCarty, K.S., Jr.; Miller, L.S.; Cox, E.B.; Konrath, J.; McCarty, K.S., Sr. Estrogen receptor analyses. Correlation of biochemical and immunohistochemical methods using monoclonal antireceptor antibodies. *Arch. Pathol. Lab. Med.* **1985**, *109*, 716–721. [PubMed]
24. Langston, C.; Kaplan, C.; Macpherson, T.; Manci, E.; Peevy, K.; Clark, B.; Murtagh, C.; Cox, S.; Glenn, G. Practice guideline for examination of the placenta: Developed by the Placental Pathology Practice Guideline Development Task Force of the College of American Pathologists. *Arch. Pathol. Lab. Med.* **1997**, *121*, 449–476.
25. Benhalima, K.; Van Crombrugge, P.; Moyson, C.; Verhaeghe, J.; Vandeginste, S.; Verlaenen, H.; Vercammen, C.; Maes, T.; Dufraimont, E.; De Block, C.; et al. Risk factor screening for gestational diabetes mellitus based on the 2013 WHO criteria. *Eur. J. Endocrinol.* **2019**, *180*, 353–363. [CrossRef] [PubMed]
26. Subiabre, M.; Silva, L.; Villalobos-Labra, R.; Toledo, F.; Paublo, M.; Lopez, M.A.; Salsoso, R.; Pardo, F.; Leiva, A.; Sobrevia, L. Maternal insulin therapy does not restore foetoplacental endothelial dysfunction in gestational diabetes mellitus. *Biochim. Biophys. Acta Mol. Basis Dis.* **2017**, *1863*, 2987–2998. [CrossRef]
27. Farias, M.; San Martin, R.; Puebla, C.; Pearson, J.D.; Casado, J.F.; Pastor-Anglada, M.; Casanello, P.; Sobrevia, L. Nitric oxide reduces adenosine transporter ENT1 gene (SLC29A1) promoter activity in human fetal endothelium from gestational diabetes. *J. Cell. Physiol.* **2006**, *208*, 451–460. [CrossRef] [PubMed]
28. Casanello, P.; Escudero, C.; Sobrevia, L. Equilibrative nucleoside (ENTs) and cationic amino acid (CATs) transporters: Implications in foetal endothelial dysfunction in human pregnancy diseases. *Curr. Vasc. Pharmacol.* **2007**, *5*, 69–84. [CrossRef] [PubMed]
29. Westermeier, F.; Puebla, C.; Vega, J.L.; Farias, M.; Escudero, C.; Casanello, P.; Sobrevia, L. Equilibrative nucleoside transporters in fetal endothelial dysfunction in diabetes mellitus and hyperglycaemia. *Curr. Vasc. Pharmacol.* **2009**, *7*, 435–449. [CrossRef]
30. da Silva, C.G.; Jarzyna, R.; Specht, A.; Kaczmarek, E. Extracellular nucleotides and adenosine independently activate AMP-activated protein kinase in endothelial cells: Involvement of P2 receptors and adenosine transporters. *Circ. Res.* **2006**, *98*, e39–e47. [CrossRef]
31. Coade, S.B.; Pearson, J.D. Metabolism of adenine nucleotides in human blood. *Circ. Res.* **1989**, *65*, 531–537. [CrossRef]
32. Yoneyama, Y.; Sawa, R.; Suzuki, S.; Ishino, H.; Miura, A.; Kuwabara, Y.; Kuwajima, T.; Ito, N.; Kiyokawa, Y.; Otsubo, Y.; et al. Regulation of plasma adenosine levels in normal pregnancy. *Gynecol. Obs. Investig.* **2002**, *53*, 71–74. [CrossRef]

33. Pardo, F.; Arroyo, P.; Salomon, C.; Westermeier, F.; Salsoso, R.; Saez, T.; Guzman-Gutierrez, E.; Leiva, A.; Sobrevia, L. Role of equilibrative adenosine transporters and adenosine receptors as modulators of the human placental endothelium in gestational diabetes mellitus. *Placenta* **2013**, *34*, 1121–1127. [CrossRef] [PubMed]
34. Salomon, C.; Westermeier, F.; Puebla, C.; Arroyo, P.; Guzman-Gutierrez, E.; Pardo, F.; Leiva, A.; Casanello, P.; Sobrevia, L. Gestational diabetes reduces adenosine transport in human placental microvascular endothelium, an effect reversed by insulin. *PLoS ONE* **2012**, *7*, e40578. [CrossRef] [PubMed]
35. Vasquez, G.; Sanhueza, F.; Vasquez, R.; Gonzalez, M.; San Martin, R.; Casanello, P.; Sobrevia, L. Role of adenosine transport in gestational diabetes-induced L-arginine transport and nitric oxide synthesis in human umbilical vein endothelium. *J. Physiol.* **2004**, *560*, 111–122. [CrossRef]
36. Higgins, M.F.; Russell, N.M.; Mooney, E.E.; McAuliffe, F.M. Clinical and ultrasound features of placental maturation in pre-gestational diabetic pregnancy. *Early Hum. Dev.* **2012**, *88*, 817–821. [CrossRef] [PubMed]
37. Huynh, J.; Dawson, D.; Roberts, D.; Bentley-Lewis, R. A systematic review of placental pathology in maternal diabetes mellitus. *Placenta* **2015**, *36*, 101–114. [CrossRef] [PubMed]
38. Evers, I.M.; Nikkels, P.G.; Sikkema, J.M.; Visser, G.H. Placental pathology in women with type 1 diabetes and in a control group with normal and large-for-gestational-age infants. *Placenta* **2003**, *24*, 819–825. [CrossRef] [PubMed]

Disclaimer/Publisher's Note: The statements, opinions and data contained in all publications are solely those of the individual author(s) and contributor(s) and not of MDPI and/or the editor(s). MDPI and/or the editor(s) disclaim responsibility for any injury to people or property resulting from any ideas, methods, instructions or products referred to in the content.

Case Report

Complete Hydatidiform Mole with Lung Metastasis and Coexisting Live Fetus: Unexpected Twin Pregnancy Mimicking Placenta Accreta

Hera Jung

Department of Pathology, CHA Ilsan Medical Center, CHA University School of Medicine, Goyang 10414, Republic of Korea; elledriver2008@gmail.com

Abstract: Twin pregnancy with a complete hydatidiform mole and coexisting fetus (CHMCF) is an exceedingly rare condition with an incidence of about 1 in 20,000–100,000 pregnancies. It can be detected by prenatal ultrasonography and an elevated maternal serum beta-human chorionic gonadotropin (BhCG) level. Herein, the author reports a case of CHMCF which was incidentally diagnosed through pathologic examination without preoperative knowledge. The 41-year-old woman, transferred due to preterm labor, delivered a female baby by cesarean section at 28 + 5 weeks of gestation. Clinically, the surgeon suspected placenta accreta on the surgical field, and the placental specimen was sent to the pathology department. On gross examination, focal vesicular and cystic lesions were identified separately from the normal-looking placental tissue. The pathologic diagnosis was CHMCF and considering the fact that placenta accreta was originally suspected, invasive hydatidiform mole was not ruled out. After radiologic work-up, metastatic lung lesions were detected, and methotrexate was administered in six cycles at intervals of every two weeks. The author presents the clinicopathological features of this unexpected CHMCF case accompanied by pulmonary metastasis, compares to literature review findings, and emphasizes the meticulous pathologic examination.

Keywords: complete hydatidiform mole; gestational trophoblastic disease; twin pregnancy

1. Introduction

Complete hydatidiform mole (CHM) is one of the gestational trophoblastic diseases originating from fertilization of an empty ovum by a sperm and can be invasive or metastatic [1]. In the early stage of CHM, clinical presentations including vaginal bleeding and a snowstorm appearance of the ultrasound lead to the detection of the disease [2]. Additionally, maternal serum beta-human chorionic gonadotropin (BhCG) level elevation also assists the prenatal diagnosis [2]. Of itself, CHM does not have the fetal part; however, twin pregnancy with a complete hydatidiform mole and a coexisting fetus (CHMCF) has been documented in about 1 in 20,000–100,000 pregnancies and the precise diagnosis of CHMCF can be delayed [3]. Herein, the author reports a case of unexpected CHMCF referred to the pathology department with a clinical impression of placenta accreta in a preterm labor.

2. Case Presentation

A 41-year-old G3-P1 multigravida woman, with 28 weeks and 4 days of gestation, was admitted to the author's institution because of preterm labor and a need for treatment in the neonatal intensive care unit (NICU). The patient had an obstetric history of dilatation and evacuation due to spontaneous abortion 4 years previously at GA (gestational age) 11 weeks, and 3 years previously she delivered a female baby weighing 3.2 kg at GA 41 weeks. The transfer record from an outside hospital presented a low-lying placenta with a suspicion of abruption and pelvic examination result of 3 cm and 50% effacement.

In the first ultrasonographic finding of the present institute, the fetus was small for the gestational age (27 + 3 weeks, 5.6 percentile) and due to the fetal position, the heart and extremities were not checked. Along with the low-lying placenta, hypervascularity and high blood flow in the subplacental area to the uterine fundus were identified. Other findings also included bridging vessels and multiple irregular lacunae within the placenta in the color Doppler ultrasound. The previous history of evacuation, maternal age, and ultrasonographic findings suggested the possibility of placenta accreta or placenta increta (Figure 1A). Moreover, there was a 4.4 cm × 3.2 cm × 2.5 cm sized mixed echoic lesion in the cervical canal, and a blood clot was suspected (Figure 1B).

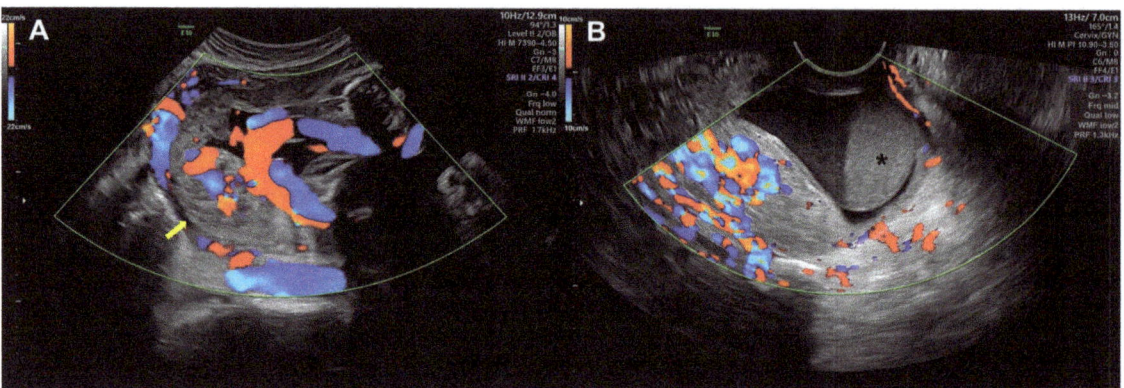

Figure 1. Ultrasonographic findings after admission. (**A**) Placenta with hypervascularity and high blood flow in subplacental area (yellow arrow); (**B**) Blood clot in cervical canal (asterisk).

After removing the blood clot with a speculum, the membrane bulged, and the length of the cervix became 0 cm with U-shaped funneling. Although magnesium sulfate (Magnesin) and ritodrine (Lavopa) were administrated, labor pain persisted every 5 to 8 min with 30–80 torr. As ultrasound findings suggested placenta accreta, the obstetrician obtained informed consent for cesarean section with the possibility of uterine artery embolization and hysterectomy in case of excessive bleeding. An emergent cesarean section was conducted on the day after admission (at GA 28 + 5 weeks). On the surgical field, the uterus was slightly dextrorotated and enlarged to term size. Bilateral ovaries and fallopian tubes were grossly normal in size and shape. The clear amniotic fluid was noted. A living female baby weighing 1030 gm with an Apgar score of 7 (at 1 min) and 8 (at 5 min) was delivered in the left occiput transverse position. Intraoperatively, the uterus showed no obvious distension over the placental bed and the surface was clear without gross neovascularity. After an initial trial of manual removal of the mildly adherent placenta, bleeding was present but controlled after an intravenous Pitocin (10 unit) injection. Therefore, no further procedure was initiated. Although the operative findings were not fully sufficient for a placenta accreta spectrum (PAS) diagnosis, the preoperative ultrasound and the experienced clinician's suspicion did not exclude placenta accreta, so the specimen was sent to the pathology department. The patient tolerated the entire procedure well and recovered in a stable condition. On gross examination at the pathology department, the placental specimen consisted of a discoid-shaped placental tissue, weighing 728 gm and measuring 23 cm × 16 cm × 2 cm. The umbilical cord inserted centrally 5 cm apart from the nearest margin and was measured 35 cm in length and 2.2 cm in diameter. On section, it had two arteries and one vein. The amniotic membrane was semitransparent. The fetal surface of the chorionic plate was smooth and semitransparent. The maternal surface was covered by intact cotyledons with blood clots and there were also separated multiple fragments of vesicular tissue, measuring up to 13 cm × 11 cm in aggregates (Figure 2A). Considering the heterogeneous gross findings and clinical suspicion of placenta accreta, sections were obtained at variable portions of the specimen. Microscopic examination demonstrated two distinct areas of villi: (1) hydropic large villi with peripheral trophoblastic hyperplasia and cistern formation; and (2) relatively small normal villi (Figure 2B). The areas of hydropic villi had massive necrotic changes, more than about 80%, and in the viable area, the enlarged villi had an internal cistern formation and circumferential trophoblast hyperplasia with often cytologic atypia (Figure 2C). Villous stromal cells and cytotrophoblasts of hydropic villi area were negative for p57 immunohistochemical staining, the marker for the maternally expressed gene CDKN1C (p57KIP2) (Figure 2D). The histologic and immunohistochemical results were consistent with complete hydatidiform mole. Meanwhile, p57 showed retained expression in normal-looking villi (Figure 2E) and there was multiple defined proliferation of capillary vessels with surface trophoblastic proliferation, consistent with choriangiomas (Figure 2F). The size of the largest choriangioma was measured to 0.5 cm. These whole pathologic findings indicated an unexpected twin pregnancy with CHMCF.

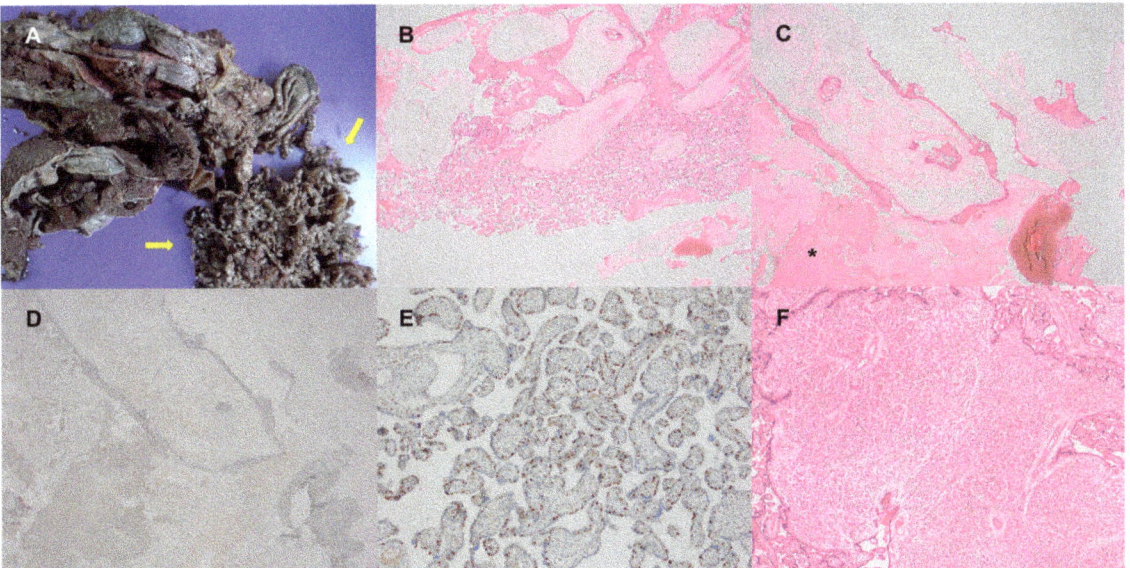

Figure 2. Gross and microscopic findings of CHMCF. (**A**) Separately identified small vesicles on gross examination (yellow arrow); (**B**) Two groups of villi: hydropic villi with cistern formation and relatively small normal-looking villi (12.5×); (**C**) Complete hydatidiform mole area with massive necrosis (asterisk) (12.5×); (**D**) Negative p57 immunohistochemical staining of complete hydatidiform mole (12.5×); (**E**) Positive p57 immunohistochemical staining of normal area (100×); (**F**) Choriangioma (40×).

Because the placenta was removed manually during surgery, there was no clear distinctive border. Additionally, the surgeon originally suspected placenta accreta and only placenta was sent for pathologic examination without any uterine tissue, so the possibility of invasive hydatidiform mole was not excluded in the clinical context. The final pathologic report was twin pregnancy with CHMCF and indicated the possibility of invasive hydatidiform mole, so a BhCG level check and radiological work-up for excluding residual or metastasizing lesions were recommended. The BhCG level at 15 days after delivery was 1325 mIU/mL. There was no previous BhCG data because an emergent section was performed. Chest computed tomography (CT) revealed variably sized nodules in both lungs, indicating hematogenous metastasis (Figure 3). Brain CT was normal and abdominopelvic CT showed postpartum uterine enlargement, fatty liver, and borderline hepatosplenomegaly.

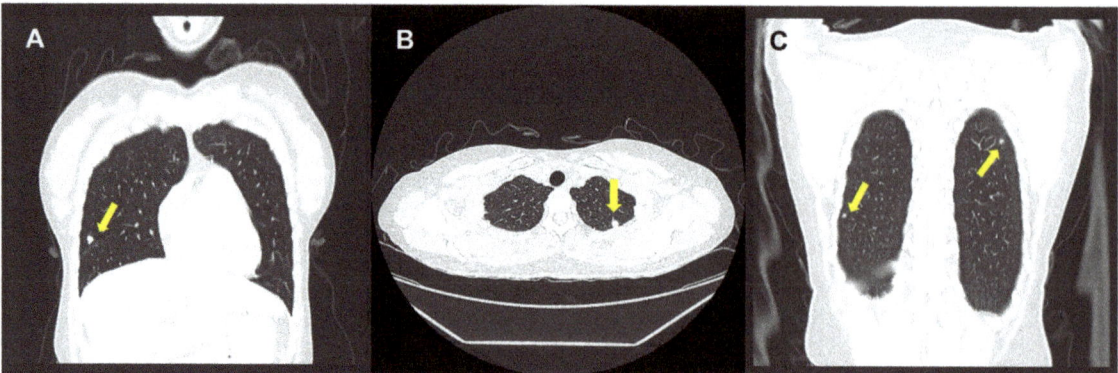

Figure 3. Chest computed tomography (CT) highlighting multiple pulmonary metastasis (yellow arrows). (**A**) Metastatic lesion in right middle lobe on coronal view; (**B**) Metastatic lesion in left upper lobe on axial view; (**C**) Metastatic lesions in both lobes on coronal view.

Six cycles of methotrexate injection were administered every two weeks. After each cycle, the BhCG level gradually decreased (399–33.9–7.2–2.4–1.2–0.4 mIU/mL). The last BhCG level was 0.2 mIU/mL at five months after delivery and follow-up CT confirmed no evidence of recurrence or metastasis in the chest and abdominopelvic cavity. The preterm baby had respiratory distress syndrome but improved and was discharged with a 2260 gm weight after two months of NICU care.

3. Discussion

Gestational trophoblastic disease is categorized by putative trophoblastic cells of placental origin; chorionic villous trophoblasts and intermediate trophoblasts [1]. Of them, hydatidiform mole originates from chorionic villous trophoblasts and is divided into complete, partial, and invasive types [1]. Among them, the pathogenesis of CHM is associated with the presence of a paternal-only genome [1]. The majority (about 80–90%) of cases are caused by duplication of the paternal haploid genome, detected as genome-wide homozygosity (46, XX), and the rest are produced by dispermy, resulting in heterozygosity (46, XX or 46, XY) [1,4]. Rarely, inherited mutation of NLRP7 or KHDC3L have also been identified as causes of familial biparental CHM [1]. Overexpression of the paternal genome leads to failure of normally balanced placental and fetal development [4]. As a result, on microscopic examination, CHM is characterized by enlarged chorionic villi with a cistern formation. Circumferential trophoblastic hyperplasia with cytologic atypia is also a usual finding and p57 immunohistochemical staining is negative in villous stromal cells and cytotrophoblasts. In CHM, fetal parts are normally absent. However, CHMCF cases have been steadily reported with low prevalence (1/20,000–100,000) [3,5–12]. The median gestational age at diagnosis of CHMCF is 15–16 weeks, and the delivery or termination is performed in 21–24 weeks [3,9]. Clinical symptoms include vaginal hemorrhage, preeclampsia, and hyperthyroidism [3]. According to the largest review article of CHMCF by M. Suksai et al., more than half of patients (118/206, 57.28%) have hemorrhage and initial BhCG levels range from 1048 to 2,460,000 mIU/mL with a median level of 367,747 mIU/mL [9]. Ultrasonography can also help the diagnosis, demonstrating snowstorm appearance and a heterogeneous, echogenic mass with cystic appearance [13]. Despite the traditional recommendation for termination of the pregnancy, several studies suggests that the risk of gestational trophoblastic neoplasia after CHMCF is not significantly increased with continuation of the pregnancy [9,10]. M. Suksai et al. reported that 37.86 % (78 of 206) were delivered successfully compared to 22.33% (46 of 203) of miscarriage or intrauterine fetal death, stillbirth, and neonatal death [9]. A better prognosis is statistically associated with the lower prevalence of antenatal maternal complications, such as pregnancy-induced hypertension (PIH), hyperthyroidism (HTD), and hyperemesis gravidarum (HG) [9]. An initial serum BhCG level less than 400,000 mIU/mL is also known as a favorable predictive factor for live births [9].

In the present case, the patient had not been diagnosed with CHMCF before and there was no serum BhCG results due to emergent admission. However, the absence of PIH, HTD, and HG might have contributed to the successful delivery. Placenta accreta was the initial clinical impression when the placental specimen was referred to the pathology department. Distinct vesicular tissues were observed on gross examination by the pathologist, so the hidden molar pregnancy obscured by a normal living fetus could be properly diagnosed. In this pregnancy, the patient was confirmed to be pregnant while living abroad but had entered South Korea during the second trimester due to the COVID-19 pandemic (patient's delivery date: 9 May 2022). The limitations on hospital visits during the pandemic period of COVID-19 are considered as a possible explanation for the delay in the diagnosis of CHMCF. The significant amount of necrosis might also be another factor that made prenatal diagnosis difficult [14]. Meanwhile, the incidence of chorangioma is 1% and associated with an increased risk of pregnancy complications, including polyhydramnios and preterm delivery [15]. Known risk factors of chorangioma include a maternal age over 30 years, maternal hypertension, twin pregnancy, maternal smoking history, and living at high altitude [15]. In the present case, the placenta of the normal living fetus had multiple chorangiomas, and two factors (maternal age and twin pregnancy) might have contributed to the development of the tumors. As multiple chorangiomas can have some overlapping ultrasonographic findings with molar pregnancy, cautious radiologic reading is also required [15]. Clinically, degenerating molar tissue can mimic placenta accreta [7]. In this case, the clinician's suspicion of placenta accreta helped the pathologic diagnosis of CHMCF with a possible invasive or metastasizing lesion. As a result, metastatic lesions that might have been missed were found, and the patient had effective chemotherapy. A lack of previous hospital information including ultrasonography and initial serum BhCG was a limitation in this case.

Additionally, the author attempted to compare this case with previous reports of CHMCF with lung metastasis. The Medline database was thoroughly searched using the PubMed retrieval service. The keywords used were "complete hydatidiform mole and surviving coexistent twin", "complete hydatidiform mole twin metastasis", "complete mole twin lung", "complete mole twin pulmonary", "complete mole fetus lung", and "complete mole fetus pulmonary". Among the studies, the cases without English publication were excluded. A total of 20 cases were collected, as those with an unspecified metastasis site and limited clinical information were omitted. Including the presented case, the clinical information from the 21 cases is displayed in Table 1. The median maternal age was 34 years. Some pregnancies were achieved by IVF (in vitro fertilization) (3 cases), hMG/hCG (human menopausal gonadotropin/human chorionic gonadotropin) therapy (1 case), and ICSI (intracytoplasmic sperm injection) (1 case). Most of the collected cases were diagnosed by prenatal BhCG or radiologic examination. Only one case in 1982 was diagnosed on delivery [16]. Thirteen cases attempted delivery including cesarean section, but in two cases, the infants died within a few hours. The detection of pulmonary metastasis was usually made after termination/delivery. Only four cases were detected before delivery at a mean GA of 25 weeks (17–32 weeks). Compared to the previous studies, the present case demonstrates the importance of pathologic examination. In most of the cases, coexisting complete hydatidiform mole was recognized in the first or second trimester, unlike this case. It is exceptional that the hidden complete hydatidiform mole and multiple lung metastases that could be harmful to the patient were diagnosed through the accurate pathological examination.

Table 1. Literature review of CHMCF with lung metastasis (21 cases).

Author (Year Published)	Maternal Age (years)	Pregnancy Type	GA at Diagnosis	BhCG Level at Diagnosis	Radiologic Finding of Complete Hydatidiform Mole	Detection of Pulmonary Metastasis	Pregnancy Outcome
Block and Merrill (1982) [16]	36	NS	On delivery	NS	Not obtained	Post OP	Amniotomy and delivery at 35 weeks
Jinno (1994) [17]	35	IVF	12 weeks	256,000 mIU/mL	Multiple cystic echoes	GA 17 weeks	Emergent cesarean section at 31 weeks (Infant died 4 h postpartum)
Osada (1995) [18]	30	Natural conception	24 weeks	478,000 mIU/mL	Typical molar pregnancy (four fifths)	7 weeks after delivery	Intrauterine fetal death and evacuation at 25 weeks
Ishii (1998) [19]	37	Natural conception	22 weeks	NS	NS	NS	Vaginal delivery at 40 weeks
Bruchium (2000) [20]	25	hMG/hCG	NS	35 MOM	Uterine wall mass	Post OP	Cesarean section at 26 weeks
Kashimura (2001) [21]	30	NS	13 weeks	684 ng/mL	Empty gestational sac with microcystic pattern	5 weeks after termination	Dilatation and evacuation (Termination)
Steigrad (2004) [22]	NS	NS	First trimester	NS	NS	Post OP	Cesarean section
Makary (2010) [23]	19	NS	25 weeks	228,000 mIU/mL	Large cystic mass	2 months after delivery	Emergent cesarean section at 25 weeks
Lee (2010) [24]	39	IVF-ET	13 weeks	1,307,693 mIU/mL	Diffuse vesicular pattern	Post OP	Hysterostomy (Termination)
Sasaki (2012) [8]	36	NS	15 weeks	440,000 mIU/mL	Typical classic molar pattern	GA 32 weeks	Spontaneous labor at 33 weeks
Sanchez-Ferrer (2013) [25]	28	Natural conception	11 weeks	395,000 mIU/mL	Multiple small cysts and a characteristic snowstorm pattern	Post OP	Suction curettage (Termination) at 13 weeks
Sanchez-Ferrer (2014) [26]	35	Natural conception	First trimester	963,971 mIU/mL	Mass of vesicular structures with snowstorm pattern	Post OP	Subtotal hysterectomy at 15 weeks (Termination and uterine rupture)

Table 1. Cont.

Author (Year Published)	Maternal Age (years)	Pregnancy Type	GA at Diagnosis	BhCG Level at Diagnosis	Radiologic Finding of Complete Hydatidiform Mole	Detection of Pulmonary Metastasis	Pregnancy Outcome
Peng (2014) [27]	34	NS	20 weeks	31,0277.7 mIU/mL	Multiple cystic spaces	4 months after delivery	Cesarean section at 37 weeks
Himoto (2014) [28]	34	Natural conception	9 weeks	1,124,200 mIU/mL	Multicystic lesion	Post OP	Artificial abortion (Termination)
Maeda (2018) [29]	33	NS	24 weeks	156,800 mIU/mL	Multicystic lesions	GA 29 weeks	Cesarean section and hysterectomy at 31 weeks
Nobuhara (2018) [30]	42	IVF	45 days	450,000 mIU/mL	Subchorionic hematoma with multivesicular features	5 weeks after termination	Aspiration curettage at 9 weeks (Termination) and delayed hysterectomy
Odera (2019) [11]	34	NS	14 weeks	900,000 mIU/mL	Mixed cystic and solid lesion with internal vascularity	GA 23 weeks	Cesarean section at 23 weeks (Infant died a few hours postpartum)
Sindiani (2020) [31]	33	NS	13 weeks	171,820 mIU/mL	A sac filled with a complete molar pregnancy	Post OP	Hysterostomy (Termination)
Mok (2021) [32]	34	NS	10 weeks	free: 13.225 MoM	Multiple cystic area	Post OP	Emergent cesarean section at 32 weeks
Alpay (2021) [33]	33	ICSI	12 weeks	425,000 mIU/mL	Echogenic mass resembling molar placenta	8 weeks after delivery	Cesarean section at 26 weeks
Jung (2023) [This work]	41	Natural conception	Not done	NS	Not identified	Post OP	Cesarean section at 28 weeks

GA: gestational age, BhCG: beta-human chorionic gonadotropin, NS: not specified, hMG/hCG: human menopausal gonadotropin/human chorionic gonadotropin, IVF: in vitro fertilization, MoM: multiples of median, ET: embryo transfer, ICSI: intracytoplasmic sperm injection.

4. Conclusions

In summary, an unexpected twin pregnancy with CHMCF and extrauterine metastasis which were clinically mimicking placenta accreta is reported. Such uncommon cases can be detected by pathological examinations, so it should always be conducted out of caution even for usual specimens. Furthermore, if placenta accreta is suspected, it is worth considering a serum BhCG check when only limited clinical information is available, such as in this case.

Funding: This research received no external funding.

Institutional Review Board Statement: This study was approved by the Institutional Review Board of CHA Ilsan Medical Center (protocol code: 2022-07-003; date of approval: 25 July 2022) with a waiver of informed consent.

Informed Consent Statement: Regarding the retrospective nature of this study, the Institutional Review Board waived the requirement for the investigator to obtain signed informed consent.

Data Availability Statement: All data are contained within the article.

Conflicts of Interest: The author declares no conflict of interest.

References

1. WHO Classification of Tumours Editorial Board. *Female Genital Tumours*; International Agency for Research on Cancer: Lyon, France, 2020.
2. Seckl, M.J.; Sebire, N.J.; Berkowitz, R.S. Gestational trophoblastic disease. *Lancet* **2010**, *376*, 717–729. [CrossRef]
3. Lin, L.H.; Maestá, I.; Braga, A.; Sun, S.Y.; Fushida, K.; Francisco, R.P.V.; Elias, K.M.; Horowitz, N.; Goldstein, D.P.; Berkowitz, R.S. Multiple pregnancies with complete mole and coexisting normal fetus in North and South America: A retrospective multicenter cohort and literature review. *Gynecol. Oncol.* **2017**, *145*, 88–95. [CrossRef] [PubMed]
4. Redline, R.W.; Boyd, T.K.; Roberts, D.J. *Placental and Gestational Pathology*; Cambridge University Press: Cambridge, UK, 2017.
5. Bristow, R.E.; Shumway, J.B.; Khouzami, A.N.; Witter, F.R. Complete hydatidiform mole and surviving coexistent twin. *Obstet. Gynecol. Surv.* **1996**, *51*, 705–709. [CrossRef] [PubMed]
6. Vaisbuch, E.; Ben-Arie, A.; Dgani, R.; Perlman, S.; Sokolovsky, N.; Hagay, Z. Twin pregnancy consisting of a complete hydatidiform mole and co-existent fetus: Report of two cases and review of literature. *Gynecol. Oncol.* **2005**, *98*, 19–23. [CrossRef]
7. Aguilera, M.; Rauk, P.; Ghebre, R.; Ramin, K. Complete hydatidiform mole presenting as a placenta accreta in a twin pregnancy with a coexisting normal fetus: Case report. *Case Rep. Obstet. Gynecol.* **2012**, *2012*, 405085. [CrossRef]
8. Sasaki, Y.; Ogawa, K.; Takahashi, J.; Okai, T. Complete hydatidiform mole coexisting with a normal fetus delivered at 33 weeks of gestation and involving maternal lung metastasis: A case report. *J. Reprod. Med.* **2012**, *57*, 301–304.
9. Suksai, M.; Suwanrath, C.; Kor-Anantakul, O.; Geater, A.; Hanprasertpong, T.; Atjimakul, T.; Pichatechaiyoot, A. Complete hydatidiform mole with co-existing fetus: Predictors of live birth. *Eur. J. Obstet. Gynecol. Reprod. Biol.* **2017**, *212*, 1–8. [CrossRef]
10. Johnson, C.; Davitt, C.; Harrison, R.; Cruz, M. Expectant Management of a Twin Pregnancy with Complete Hydatidiform Mole and Coexistent Normal Fetus. *Case Rep. Obstet. Gynecol.* **2019**, *2019*, 8737080. [CrossRef]
11. Odedra, D.; MacEachern, K.; Elit, L.; Mohamed, S.; McCready, E.; DeFrance, B.; Wang, Y. Twin pregnancy with metastatic complete molar pregnancy and coexisting live fetus. *Radiol. Case Rep.* **2020**, *15*, 195–200. [CrossRef]
12. Tipiani Rodríguez, O.; Solís Sosa, C.; Valdez Alegría, G.E.; Quenaya Rodríguez, R.J.; Escalante Jibaja, R.; Cevallos Pacheco, C.; Ibarra Lavado, O.; Bocanegra Becerra, Y.L. Invasive hydatidiform mole coexistent with normal fetus. Case report. *Rev. Peru. Ginecol. Obstet.* **2020**, *66*, 1–5. [CrossRef]
13. Green, C.L.; Angtuaco, T.L.; Shah, H.R.; Parmley, T.H. Gestational trophoblastic disease: A spectrum of radiologic diagnosis. *RadioGraphics* **1996**, *16*, 1371–1384. [CrossRef] [PubMed]
14. Okumura, M.; Fushida, K.; Francisco, R.P.V.; Schultz, R.; Zugaib, M. Massive Necrosis of a Complete Hydatidiform Mole in a Twin Pregnancy With a Surviving Coexistent Fetus. *J. Ultrasound Med.* **2014**, *33*, 177–179. [CrossRef] [PubMed]
15. Akbarzadeh-Jahromi, M.; Soleimani, N.; Mohammadzadeh, S. Multiple Chorangioma Following Long-Term Secondary Infertility: A Rare Case Report and Review of Pathologic Differential Diagnosis. *Int. Med. Case Rep. J.* **2019**, *12*, 383–387. [CrossRef] [PubMed]
16. Block, M.F.; Merrill, J.A. Hydatidiform mole with coexistent fetus. *Obstet. Gynecol.* **1982**, *60*, 129–133. [PubMed]
17. Jinno, M.; Ubukata, Y.; Hanyu, I.; Satou, M.; Yoshimura, Y.; Nakamura, Y. Hydatidiform mole with a surviving coexisting fetus following in-vitro fertilization. *Hum. Reprod.* **1994**, *9*, 1770–1772. [CrossRef]
18. Osada, H.; Iitsuka, Y.; Matsui, H.; Sekiya, S. A Complete Hydatidiform Mole Coexisting with a Normal Fetus Was Confirmed by Variable Number Tandem Repeat (VNTR) Polymorphism Analysis Using Polymerase Chain Reaction. *Gynecol. Oncol.* **1995**, *56*, 90–93. [CrossRef]
19. Ishii, J.; Iitsuka, Y.; Takano, H.; Matsui, H.; Osada, H.; Sekiya, S. Genetic differentiation of complete hydatidiform moles coexisting with normal fetuses by short tandem repeat–derived deoxyribonucleic acid polymorphism analysis. *Am. J. Obstet. Gynecol.* **1998**, *179*, 628–634. [CrossRef]
20. Bruchim, I.; Kidron, D.; Amiel, A.; Altaras, M.; Fejgin, M.D. Complete Hydatidiform Mole and a Coexistent Viable Fetus: Report of Two Cases and Review of the Literature. *Gynecol. Oncol.* **2000**, *77*, 197–202. [CrossRef]
21. Kashimura, Y.; Tanaka, M.; Harada, N.; Shinmoto, M.; Morishita, T.; Morishita, H.; Kashimura, M. Twin pregnancy consisting of 46, XY heterozygous complete mole coexisting with a live fetus. *Placenta* **2001**, *22*, 323–327. [CrossRef]
22. Steigrad, S.J.; Robertson, G.; Kaye, A.L. Serial hCG and ultrasound measurements for predicting malignant potential in multiple pregnancies associated with complete hydatidiform mole: A report of 2 cases. *J. Reprod. Med.* **2004**, *49*, 554–558.
23. Makary, R.; Mohammadi, A.; Rosa, M.; Shuja, S. Twin gestation with complete hydatidiform mole and a coexisting live fetus: Case report and brief review of literature. *Obstet. Med.* **2010**, *3*, 30–32. [CrossRef] [PubMed]

24. Lee, S.W.; Kim, M.Y.; Chung, J.H.; Yang, J.H.; Lee, Y.H.; Chun, Y.K. Clinical findings of multiple pregnancy with a complete hydatidiform mole and coexisting fetus. *J. Ultrasound Med.* **2010**, *29*, 271–280. [CrossRef] [PubMed]
25. Sánchez-Ferrer, M.L.; Machado-Linde, F.; Martínez-Espejo Cerezo, A.; Peñalver Parres, C.; Ferri, B.; López-Expósito, I.; Abad, L.; Parrilla, J.J. Management of a Dichorionic Twin Pregnancy with a Normal Fetus and an Androgenetic Diploid Complete Hydatidiform Mole. *Fetal Diagn. Ther.* **2013**, *33*, 194–200. [CrossRef] [PubMed]
26. Sánchez-Ferrer, M.L.; Hernández-Martínez, F.; Machado-Linde, F.; Ferri, B.; Carbonel, P.; Nieto-Diaz, A. Uterine rupture in twin pregnancy with normal fetus and complete hydatidiform mole. *Gynecol. Obstet. Investig.* **2014**, *77*, 127–133. [CrossRef] [PubMed]
27. Peng, H.H.; Huang, K.G.; Chueh, H.Y.; Adlan, A.S.; Chang, S.D.; Lee, C.L. Term delivery of a complete hydatidiform mole with a coexisting living fetus followed by successful treatment of maternal metastatic gestational trophoblastic disease. *Taiwan. J. Obstet. Gynecol.* **2014**, *53*, 397–400. [CrossRef]
28. Himoto, Y.; Kido, A.; Minamiguchi, S.; Moribata, Y.; Okumura, R.; Mogami, H.; Nagano, T.; Konishi, I.; Togashi, K. Prenatal differential diagnosis of complete hydatidiform mole with a twin live fetus and placental mesenchymal dysplasia by magnetic resonance imaging. *J. Obstet. Gynaecol. Res.* **2014**, *40*, 1894–1900. [CrossRef]
29. Maeda, Y.; Oyama, R.; Maeda, H.; Imai, Y.; Yoshioka, S. Choriocarcinoma with multiple lung metastases from complete hydatidiform mole with coexistent fetus during pregnancy. *J. Obstet. Gynaecol. Res.* **2018**, *44*, 1476–1481. [CrossRef]
30. Nobuhara, I.; Harada, N.; Haruta, N.; Higashiura, Y.; Watanabe, H.; Watanabe, S.; Hisanaga, H.; Sado, T. Multiple metastatic gestational trophoblastic disease after a twin pregnancy with complete hydatidiform mole and coexisting fetus, following assisted reproductive technology: Case report and literature review. *Taiwan. J. Obstet. Gynecol.* **2018**, *57*, 588–593. [CrossRef]
31. Sindiani, A.; Obeidat, B.; Alshdaifat, E. Successful Management of the First Case of a Metastasized Complete Mole in Form of Twin Pregnancy in Jordan. *Am. J. Case Rep.* **2020**, *21*, e923395. [CrossRef]
32. Mok, Z.W.; Merchant, K.; Yip, S.L. Management of a complete hydatidiform mole with a coexisting live fetus followed by successful treatment of maternal metastatic gestational trophoblastic disease: Learning points. *BMJ Case Rep.* **2021**, *14*, e235028. [CrossRef]
33. Alpay, V.; Kaymak, D.; Erenel, H.; Cepni, I.; Madazli, R. Complete Hydatidiform Mole and Co-Existing Live Fetus after Intracytoplasmic Sperm Injection: A Case Report and Literature Review. *Fetal Pediatr. Pathol.* **2021**, *40*, 493–500. [CrossRef] [PubMed]

Disclaimer/Publisher's Note: The statements, opinions and data contained in all publications are solely those of the individual author(s) and contributor(s) and not of MDPI and/or the editor(s). MDPI and/or the editor(s) disclaim responsibility for any injury to people or property resulting from any ideas, methods, instructions or products referred to in the content.

MDPI
St. Alban-Anlage 66
4052 Basel
Switzerland
www.mdpi.com

Diagnostics Editorial Office
E-mail: diagnostics@mdpi.com
www.mdpi.com/journal/diagnostics

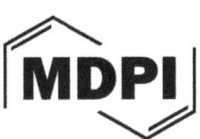

Disclaimer/Publisher's Note: The statements, opinions and data contained in all publications are solely those of the individual author(s) and contributor(s) and not of MDPI and/or the editor(s). MDPI and/or the editor(s) disclaim responsibility for any injury to people or property resulting from any ideas, methods, instructions or products referred to in the content.

www.ingramcontent.com/pod-product-compliance
Lightning Source LLC
LaVergne TN
LVHW070600100526
838202LV00012B/526